Personalisation and Dementia

A Guide for Person-Centred Practice

HELEN SANDERSON AND GILL BAILEY

FOREWORD BY JEREMY HUGHES

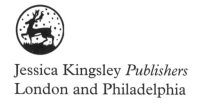
Jessica Kingsley *Publishers*
London and Philadelphia

First published in 2014
by Jessica Kingsley Publishers
73 Collier Street
London N1 9BE, UK
and
400 Market Street, Suite 400
Philadelphia, PA 19106, USA

www.jkp.com

Library of Congress Cataloging in Publication Data
A CIP catalog record for this book is available from the Library of Congress

British Library Cataloguing in Publication Data
A CIP catalogue record for this book is available from the British Library

ISBN 978 1 84905 379 2
eISBN 978 0 85700 734 6

Printed and bound in Great Britain by Bell & Bain Ltd, Glasgow

Personalisation
and Dementia

by the same author

Creating Person-Centred Organisations
Strategies and Tools for Managing Change in Health, Social Care and the Voluntary Sector
Stephen Stirk and Helen Sanderson
ISBN 978 1 84905 260 3
eISBN 978 0 85700 549 6

A Practical Guide to Delivering Personalisation
Person-Centred Practice in Health and Social Care
Helen Sanderson and Jaimee Lewis
ISBN 978 1 84905 194 1
eISBN 978 0 85700 422 2

of related interest

Enriched Care Planning for People with Dementia
A Good Practice Guide to Delivering Person-Centred Care
Hazel May, Paul Edwards and Dawn Brooker
ISBN 978 1 84310 405 6
eISBN 978 1 84642 960 6
Bradford Dementia Group Good Practice Guides series

Person-Centred Dementia Care
Making Services Better
Dawn Brooker
ISBN 978 1 84310 337 0
eISBN 978 1 84642 588 2
Bradford Dementia Group Good Practice Guides series

Contents

Foreword

'Personalisation' is at the heart of what the Alzheimer's Society is working to achieve for people affected by dementia every day.

Not a 'one size fits all' service that you're expected to fit into, but a genuinely responsive approach that delivers what people want, in the way they want it, by people they want to receive it from.

It means more one-to-one conversation to establish how best to support someone and to keep having that conversation as desires and expectations change.

Great strides have been made over recent times in dementia policy and establishing dementia as a national priority. The challenge now is to use this commitment to ensure better day-to-day lived experience of people with dementia. For this, we need proven and practical approaches that deliver in practice what policy promises in principle.

People with dementia consistently tell us that they want to have choice and control over decisions about them; for services to be designed around them and their needs; and to feel a valued part of family, community and civic life.

And yet people still ask if personalisation can ever work for people with dementia. This has always struck me as the wrong question to be asking.

Instead of 'can' personalisation work, surely we need to be asking 'how' we make it work on a scale whereby it becomes the expectation of anyone seeking care and support to help them live well with dementia.

This is where I hope the latest book from Helen Sanderson and Gill Bailey will have its greatest impact.

Personalisation builds upon person centred care, with an increased focus on choice and control for the individual. This book shows how adopting person centred practices into everyday practice can make significant changes for all people, regardless of their type or stage of dementia.

At its heart, personalisation is about observing, listening and understanding what makes a person tick, what gives them hope, enjoyment and meaning in their everyday life, and then tailoring care and support to help them either attain or retain these.

The person centred practices outlined in this book show how to deliver genuine personalisation, where what is important *for* the person is balanced with what is important *to* the person's wellbeing. It is about the stuff that makes a life worth living: each person as an individual with their own needs, wishes and dreams to be recognised and met.

Excellent support and quality care has always been more than just about money and who pays for services. Personalisation needs to be delivered in across the community; including support and care in the home and in residential care too.

Personal budgets can be an effective route to personalisation but only when they deliver what a person wants; there is sufficient information and support available; and the amount of money is realistic. Again, the approaches clearly laid out in this book, if followed, will help ensure the drive towards personal budgets takes place within the context of delivering improved and tailored outcomes for individual people. In the current economic climate, it is even more important that we make sure personalisation is about real choice and service. It is not, and must not be seen as a way of cutting funding.

I therefore warmly welcome the timely publication of a book that seeks to ensure we always see the person and not the dementia.

Jeremy Hughes
Chief Executive, Alzheimer's Society

Acknowledgements

In this book we share what we are learning with and from people living with dementia. We are grateful to everyone who gave their permission for their story to be told. All names have been changed, unless people have requested that their name is used.

We are grateful to the following people for their help with this book: Kerry Buckley and Hilary Bradley for their help with the text and references; Julie Barclay for designing the figures; Jon Ralphs for the graphic history; Michelle Livesley for helping us think about the community chapter; Martin Routledge for co-authoring Chapter 2; Sally Percival for writing her story about her mum; and Alison Macadam and NDTi for sharing William's story.

Thank you to the people, staff and manager, Lisa Martin, at Bruce Lodge and the team from Stockport Council and Borough Care Limited for My Home, My Life, My Choice. Thank you also to Angela Boyle and staff at Alternative Futures Group.

Thank you to the HSA and HSA Press teams, for their support and encouragement – Charlotte Sweeney, Ruth Gorman, Michelle Livesley, Jo Harvey, Vicky Jones, Alison Short, Jon Ralphs, Kerry Buckley, Andy Gitsham, Jan Eva and Claire Ashworth.

This book builds on our earlier publications and the information shared on our websites. We have quoted from Helen Bowers and referred to material from our earlier book *Plans and Practicalities: Person-Centred Thinking with Older People* (Bowers *et al.* 2007). We have used some of the material from our work with Max Neill on circles of support.

All the stories and designed example person-centred thinking tools are shared with the permission of HSA and are also available through our websites and blogs.

The learning about person-centred practices that is shared in this book has been developed by an international community. Michael Smull is the Chair of the Learning Community for Person-Centred Practices, and Helen is Director Emeritus. Michael Smull and members of the Learning Community developed the person-centred thinking tools in this book and you can learn more about our work at www.learningcommunity.us.

For information and support on implementing person-centred practices with people living with dementia, please go to www.helensandersonassociates.co.uk, and for materials and resources, see www.hsapress.co.uk.

The appendix is *Progress for Providers*. This was developed by Samantha Leonard (Joint Commissioning Manager, Lancashire County Council and NHS Central Lancashire), Nicole Alkemade (Older People's Joint Commissioning Manager, NHS Stockport), Angela Boyle (Assistant Director, Alternative Futures Group), Carey Bamber (Associate, In Control), Trevor Adams (Founder, Passionate Dementia Care), Martin Routledge (Head of Operations, In Control), Gill Bailey (Helen Sanderson Associates) and Helen Sanderson (Director, Helen Sanderson Associates).

Chapter 1

About this Book

And Arthur

> We started using one-page profiles at Bruce Lodge a year ago. This approach has really made a difference to both staff and people who live here. I was surprised at what a big difference we have made to people, and our culture has changed from being very task-focused to thinking about people and what matters to them, and exactly how they want to be supported.
>
> *Lisa Martin, Manager, Bruce Lodge, Borough Care*

> I can't believe we are sat talking about me and things that matter to me, which I thought were gone for ever.
>
> *Mary Stuart, who lives at Bruce Lodge*

Arthur's story

Arthur is 86 and a charming man, described as the 'salt of the earth; a true character and a real gent'. He has early-onset dementia. He has lived in his own flat in an inner-city area for 35 years. He lost his wife, Madge, 20 years ago and treasures her wedding ring, which he wears on his little finger. He loves talking to people and is an amazing storyteller. Sometimes he likes to talk about his time driving tanks during the war, but only when he is in the mood. He also likes to talk about boxers from decades ago.

Arthur is supported by the local domiciliary care services. His district nurse, Marie, was concerned that Arthur may need residential care. Arthur is terrified of being 'put in a home', and Marie asked her colleague Gill Bailey to help, as Gill was familiar with person-centred practices. Gill spent an hour with Arthur, asking him about his past, what makes up a good or bad day, how he'd like to be supported and what kind of routine he enjoys. She used this to develop a one-page profile, which contained all this information. Gill then met with Arthur, his nephew Stephen and Stephen's wife, Sally, the manager of the domiciliary service and a staff member. Together, they looked at the one-page profile and talked about what was working and not working in Arthur's life from each of their perspectives.

From Arthur's perspective, the highlight of his week was spending Friday evenings with Stephen, Sally and their three children, whom he loves dearly. Stephen also phoned him at 5pm every day. Arthur felt both of these actions worked well for him. He also said it was important to have someone to talk to, especially at meal times. His staff spent their time making his meal and left it with him, but they did not have time to sit and chat. He also said it was important that his meals were served piping hot. It didn't work for him when staff gave him his dinner lukewarm and left him just a sandwich for lunch. Arthur usually threw both meals into his back yard. This caused problems with his neighbours and a rat infestation. Arthur also said he was 'sick and tired' of people telling him to take off his wool bob hat.

From the staff's perspective, it did not work when Arthur sometimes hit out with his walking stick when they came to wake him in the morning. As he can't see well, he had assumed they were burglars. Arthur's poor eyesight meant that good support would be for staff to call him from the bedroom door to wake him up, and never to approach him and shake him while he slept. Staff were also concerned that he sometimes wandered out late at night, which was not safe. They said Arthur made sense of his days by sticking to his routine. He needed to be reminded daily if something out of the ordinary was happening; otherwise he became disoriented, confused and was likely to go outdoors in search of help.

Stephen said that something that did not work for him was Arthur's late-night phone calls when he couldn't find the £10 note he usually kept in his pocket 'in case he needs it'. Some of the staff had taken this out of his pocket for 'safekeeping' and put it away in his drawer, but Arthur would become distressed looking for it, sometimes struggling on his hands and knees for hours.

Together, Arthur, his family and staff agreed some simple actions that meant that Arthur could stay living in his own home and addressed what was not working for him. Staff agreed to use the one-page profile as the way to support Arthur, particularly concerning how to help him wake up in the morning (by calling from the door) and never taking his £10 note out of his pocket. The family suggested that Sally provide frozen meals for Arthur, so that staff simply heated these until they were piping hot. They could then use their time to stay and talk to Arthur while he ate. This made life better for Arthur; he started to eat well, had company and no longer had problems with his neighbours. The staff treated the rat infestation. Arthur agreed to a mat sensor, which can be activated at night to detect when he leaves the house. These small but significant changes meant that Arthur's life improved and that staff could support him in the way that he wanted.

Arthur's story shows how understanding what is important to someone and then finding out how they want to be supported and acting exactly as they wish can make a huge difference to their life. This information was recorded on a single side of paper (called a one-page profile) after Gill spent a couple of hours talking to Arthur and meeting with his staff and family. Together, they came up with actions that addressed what was not working for everyone, which meant that staff worked with him in a different way to achieve the changes he wanted. These new ways of working represented a shift in power and a change of culture. This is personalisation, delivered through person-centred practices. Person-centred practices are simply a different way of listening that results in a different kind of action.

This book will show you what personalisation can mean in everyday practice for people living with dementia, and how to deliver this through person-centred practices. This approach builds on person-centred care and focuses on how people living with dementia can have more choice and control in their lives, and be supported to be part of their community – even if they live in residential care. We believe that person-centred practices have a vital role to play in enabling people with dementia to be heard, along with their families, and to find solutions that can change and ease people's lives, while also creating a more person-centred culture in organisations.

The book starts with a chapter co-authored by our colleague Martin Routledge, explaining what personalisation is and where person-centred practices have come from. These person-centred practices were developed by the Learning Community for Person-Centred Practices (www.learningcommunity.us) and are used with families, in education, in hospitals and health care, in social care and hospices; in fact, they can be used from birth to the end of life.

Person-centred practices enable us to:

- Learn differently about the person – about what really matters to them, from their perspective and how to deliver good support to keep people healthy, safe and well (we look at this in Chapter 3).

- Learn how the person communicates and how we can support people to make more choices and decisions (as described in Chapter 4).

- Think differently about staff and how we can match staff to people living with dementia in a way that reflects interests and personalities (we look at this and how to clarify staff roles in Chapter 5).

- Develop and act on person-centred information through the use of person-centred reviews (which we explain in Chapter 6).

- Reflect and learn more about the person and how we are delivering support using person-centred thinking tools (we describe these in Chapter 7).

- Take a fresh look at life stories, recognised as good practice in supporting people with dementia, and reflect on supporting people to think about the future (Chapter 8).

- Think about community, which is crucial to people's lives, and how we enable people to be contributing members of their community and civic life (Chapter 9).

In Chapter 10 we share a story that demonstrates how the different person-centred thinking tools can be used together and how they made a difference to John. Finally, we help you get started on this journey in Chapter 11 when we introduce the self-assessment tool called *Progress for Providers*.

In this book we share many examples of how information from person-centred thinking tools can be recorded, but fundamentally these tools are a way to have a different conversation and to act on it. Person-centred practices should not increase bureaucracy in any way. We are working with providers to demonstrate how they can reduce, and not increase, paperwork through incorporating person-centred thinking tools.

This book is not simply about a new set of tools or practices. We think it reflects a different way of thinking about people and staff, beyond life stories, to connect to what matters to people now. We have learned from and respectfully build on the work of Dawn Brooker on person-centred care, Mike Nolan on relationship-centred care and Ruth Bartlett on citizenship and community (Brooker 2007; Nolan *et al.* 2004; Bartlett and O'Connor 2010). These themes reflect the essence of where we hope person-centred practices can be used and developed in the future, in creating a new relationship between the person with dementia and paid staff, fully respecting the experience and knowledge of carers, and designing services and supports around individuals. Staying focused on people with dementia, not just in their community but making a contribution to community and civic life, is an area that is crucially important for all of us. There is so much more to learn about how to make this a reality.

A note on how this book was written

This book shares the lives and journeys of people and their families with whom we have worked directly over the last five years. There are stories from people who have early-onset dementia and who live at home with support, and from their families. You will meet Fong who lives with her husband, Tony; Louisa and Hilda who live by themselves with domiciliary care; Audree and Doris who live with their families; and Mary who lives in extra care housing.

You will meet Doreen, Edie, Ann, Olive, Meg, Saskia, Winifred, Joe, Ken, Dorothy, Annie, Bessie, Frank, Audrey, Grace, Julia, June, Marion, Betty, Pauline and John who live in a range of different-sized care homes. We have tried to get a balance between stories where people's families are involved and where people only have paid staff in their life.

Sharing these stories, with people's permission, and having quotations from people who live with dementia is the closest we could come to hearing from people who live with dementia. Helen and Gill both volunteer at a home for people living with dementia.

If you want a detailed account of person-centred practices from a more academic context, we refer you to *Progress in Personalisation for People Living with Dementia* by Adams, Routledge and Sanderson (2012). The most effective way to deliver person-centred practices is to look at culture and practices at an organisational level too. If you are interested in this, you may like to look at *Creating Person-Centred Organisations* by Stirk and Sanderson (2012). If you want to explore the ideas about community in Chapter 9, then we recommend the work of the National Development Team for Inclusion (NDTi) on circles of support for people with dementia and Inclusion Webs (www.NDTi.org.uk), and Local Area Coordination (LAC) and the work of Ralph Broad (http:// inclusiveneighbourhoods.co.uk).

Finally, we are still exploring, trying and learning about how to ensure that people with dementia have the lifestyle and support that they deserve. You can read more about this on our website www.helensandersonassociates.co.uk and blog.

Chapter 2

Personalisation and People Living with Dementia

With Martin Routledge

> Personalisation means thinking about care and support services in an entirely different way. This means starting with the person as an individual with strengths, preferences and aspirations and putting them at the centre of the process of identifying their needs and making choices about how and when they are supported to live their lives. It requires a significant transformation of adult social care so that all systems, processes, staff and services are geared up to put people first.
>
> *Social Care Institute of Excellence 2010, p.1*

Personalisation for people living with dementia means figuring out how people can have as much choice and control as possible in their day-to-day life. This means, for example, that people living in a care home are supported to decide when they want to get up, rather than this being determined by staff; when they want to have breakfast, instead of a set time for everyone; and how they want to spend their time, rather than just choosing whether to join in with a group activity in the afternoon or not.

Our ambition over the last decade has been that people are treated with dignity and respect. Personalisation raises the bar: to expect person-centred care and to take this further for people to direct their life and service as much as they can.

Personalisation was introduced into English social policy in the *Putting People First* 'concordat' (Department of Health 2007), although the push for what has become called personalisation had come from disabled people, their families and their progressive allies in public services over several decades. People increasingly want to use the resources available for their support – whether they are publicly or privately funded – in a way that is most meaningful for them, rather than accepting a 'one size fits all' approach.

At the heart of personalisation is 'self-direction' – the notion that people should not simply be passive recipients of services but should be able to exercise direction over their support, which should be designed around and with them. This self-direction will, of course, vary in terms of the levels and nature of control that people are able and wish to take, but it should not be denied to anyone, regardless of their disability or personal circumstances. Research and evaluation of personalisation show positive effects on people's lives and higher levels of satisfaction.

Personal budgets – meaning that people using social care direct the resources for their care and support – are a major element of personalisation but certainly not the only one. A personal budget sets out, after assessment, the amount of money available for a person's community-based care and support, and should allow the person and (where appropriate) those close to them to be strongly involved in deciding how that money can be used to best meet their needs. The resource can then be taken as a cash 'direct payment' or managed on the person's behalf, if they wish, by the local authority or nominated others, or held by a provider as an Individual Service Fund. Hence the person can take as much direct control as they wish and their circumstances allow over the resources for their support.

Individual Service Funds (ISF) are a mechanism for people to have control over their service. An ISF means that people have an allocation of money or time (hours), and the person decides how they want to spend this. Best practice in Individual Service Funds means that people choose what they spend their time or money on, where, who they want to support them, when they use it, and specify how they are supported. This may sound radical and impossible in a care home setting, yet we are seeing some early pioneering work, exploring how far we can go. We are learning that person-centred practices are crucial for learning 'what, how, who, when and where' and that this requires leadership and a commitment to completely rethink how staff time is used, and therefore how rotas work.

There are clear, positive impacts of personal budgets and the White Paper *Caring for Our Future: Reforming Care and Support* (HM Government 2012) announced the piloting of an extension of direct payments (the cash personal budget option) into residential care.

Think Local, Act Personal (TLAP) – a cross-sector social care partnership of central and local government, people using social care, and provider and voluntary bodies – was formed in 2011 to further promote the practical delivery of personalisation. TLAP (2011) published *Making it Real*, a set of markers of progress for personalisation developed primarily by people who use social care and family carers, reflecting the key elements of the TLAP manifesto. The markers constitute 26 clustered 'I' statements and a range of associated elements that would need to be in place within a locality or organisation to promote 'real' personalisation. These markers are supported by central and local government, the Care Quality Commission and key provider umbrella bodies, and there are links between the TLAP markers of progress in personalisation and the Dementia Action Alliance's National Dementia Declaration.

The Dementia Action Alliance is made up of over 250 organisations committed to transforming the quality of life of people living with dementia and comprises organisations that have signed the National Dementia Declaration (see www.dementiaaction.org.uk). The declaration identifies the challenge dementia represents to the UK and outlines outcomes that range from ensuring people with dementia have choice and control over their lives, to feeling a valued part of family, community and civic life, including people living with dementia having personal choice and control or influence over decisions that affect them. The key statements from the declaration are shown here.

National Dementia Declaration

1. I have personal choice and control or influence over decisions about me.

2. I know that services are designed around me and my needs.

3. I have support that helps me live my life.

4. I have the knowledge and know-how to get what I need.

5. I live in an enabling and supportive environment where I feel valued and understood.

6. I have a sense of belonging and of being a valued part of family, community and civic life.

7. I know there is research going on, which delivers a better life for me now and hope for the future.

The context for personalisation and dementia

Caring for our future: reforming care and support (2012)
White paper that announced the piloting of an extension of direct payments (the cash personal budget option) into residential care.

The Dementia Action Alliance
An alliance of over 250 organisations committed to transforming the quality of life of people living with dementia and comprises organisations that have signed the National Dementia Declaration (see www.dementiaaction.org.uk).

The National Dementia Declaration
The declaration identifies the challenge dementia represents. The declaration outlines outcomes that range from ensuring people with dementia have choice and control over their lives, to the UK and community and civic life, to feeling a valued part of family, community personal choice including people living with dementia having decisions which affect them. and control or influence over decisions which affect them.

Putting People First (2007)
Introduces personalisation

Personal Budgets
A major way to deliver personalisation. A personal budget sets out, after assessment, the amount of money available for a person's community-based care and support and should allow the person and (where appropriate) those close to them to be strongly involved in deciding how that money can be used to best meet needs. The resource can then be taken as a cash direct payment' or managed on the person's behalf, or as an Individual Service Fund with a provider.

Think Local Act Personal (TLAP)
a cross-sector social care partnership of central and local government, people using social care, and provider and voluntary bodies – formed in 2011 to further promote the practical delivery of personalisation

Making it Real
A set of markers of progress for personalisation developed primarily by people who use social care and family carers. The markers constitute 26 clustered 'I' statements that would need to be in place within a locality or organisation to promote 'real' personalisation.

Figure 2.1 The context for personalisation and dementia

Personalisation in practice

Delivering personalisation in practice for people living with dementia has been variable. Some good work has taken place in this area (see, for example, Mental Health Foundation 2011). However, it is disappointing, if not surprising, that older people and particularly people with dementia are currently not benefiting sufficiently. While there have been more than 20 years of development of effective and evidenced-based person-centred approaches, which enable greater personalisation for people using all kinds of supports and services, these approaches are far from universally applied. The purpose of this book is to make a contribution to showing how person-centred practices can deliver more personalised support for people living with dementia.

There are some emerging, encouraging examples of Individual Service Funds being introduced to people living with dementia – for example, in Bruce Lodge, a care home in Stockport. This is a partnership between the commissioners of the service, Stockport Local Authority; a provider, Borough Care Ltd; and Helen Sanderson Associates (where the work was led by the authors).

Individual Service Funds (ISF) are a mechanism for people to have control over their service and have to start with an allocation of money or time. At Bruce Lodge, home for 43 people with dementia, the provider (Borough Care) and the commissioners worked out what they could try to allocate each individual. Ideally, each person would have an individual allocation based on assessment. At Bruce Lodge, we decided that to move in that direction, each person would have an allocation of two hours a month for individual support, and we needed to find these two hours without additional funding.

The next step was to help people think about how they wanted to spend their two hours. The manager, Lisa, worked with Gill Bailey (one of the authors) to meet with the person, and their family where possible, to have a different kind of conversation based on the person-centred thinking tools that we describe in this book.

The people at Bruce Lodge are now using their personal support time in many different ways. Annie goes to Ashton market and has tea and cake or a meal there. John goes out on a boat. Bessie is making a scrapbook of her life and travels, which her daughter Barbara is helping with. Doreen used to be an assistant verger at her church and a member of the Mothers' Union and is now going to church services again. Saskia has later-stage dementia and, after thinking with her and her family, our best guess was that she would enjoy going out to the park and sitting by the bowling green to have an ice cream or to have someone read aloud to her – Danielle Steele was always a favourite author.

For more information about ISFs with people with dementia, see Sanderson and Miller (in press).

Generally, though, people with dementia are not benefiting sufficiently from services becoming more personalised or from personal budgets. One of the challenges for providers is that it can be difficult to know where to start and, sometimes, what they could be aspiring to. There are excellent evaluation processes such as Dawn Brooker's VIPS and Dementia Care Mapping (see www.bradford.ac.uk/health/career_areas/dementia-group/short-courses/dementia-care-mapping/dementia-care-mapping-data-sheets) that provide direction on delivering improved person-centred care, but there is nothing that captures what needs to be in place to deliver truly personalised services to individuals with dementia, and which looks at how the roles of managers and staff have to change to be person-centred in order to deliver person-centred services. This is what *Progress for Providers: Checking Your Progress in Delivering Personalised Support for People Living with Dementia* is trying to achieve. We introduce this in Chapter 11 of this book.

Person-centred practices to deliver personalisation

To deliver personalised services, we need to know what is important to a person, how to best support them, how they communicate and make decisions, and how we are doing in delivering personalised services – what is working and not working. This is where person-centred practices can help.

The current vision for health and adult social care requires that person-centred practice and self-directed support become mainstream activities in order to deliver personalisation (Department of Health 2008, 2010b). Person-centred practices have a strong role to play in helping people to be heard, finding solutions and changing people's lives, while also changing the culture of the organisations that provide care and support services. They include simple, effective and evidence-based practices – including person-centred thinking, person-centred reviews, person-centred planning and support planning – and are proven ways to do this (Robertson *et al.* 2005).

Person-centred thinking tools have their foundation in person-centred planning – an approach to social justice and inclusion originally developed in supporting people with learning disabilities (Sanderson and Lewis 2012). The Learning Community for Person-Centred Practices (www.learningcommunity.us) mainly developed these tools, and the foundation skill underpinning them is being able to separate what is important *to* someone, from what is important *for* them, and finding a balance between the two (Smull and Sanderson 2005). Other tools have been adapted from management practice; for example, the doughnut is taken directly from Charles Handy's 1994 work on organisational behaviour and management. Person-centred thinking tools have also been developed from the contributions of leaders in the disability inclusion movement and personalisation – for example, Beth Mount and John O'Brien.

Person-centred thinking refers to a range of practical tools and skills that staff can use on a day-to-day basis to deliver more personalised services. *Person-centred reviews* are a way to transform and replace the statutory required reviews in services to create person-centred actions. *Person-centred planning* refers to processes for planning around an individual, which focus on creating a positive future and being part of a community. *Support planning* is a way for individuals to describe what they want to change about their life and how they will use their personal budget to do so (Sanderson and Lewis 2012). The Skills for Care and Dementia UK guide *Dementia: Workers and Carers Together* (2012) recommends that providers keep up to date with best practice such as person-centred practices and approaches.

Person-centred thinking tools enable staff to deliver personalised services by helping to answer the following questions:

- How does the person want to live and be supported?

- How can the person have more choice and control in his life?

- What is our role in delivering what is important to the person and how he wants to be supported?

- How are we doing in supporting the person in the way he wants to live?

- How can we work together to keep what is working and change what is not working?

- How can we keep learning about the person and what we need to do to provide the best support?

In Figure 2.2 we show how person-centred practices can help to deliver what people affected by dementia have said they want to see in their lives (as described in the National Dementia Declaration).

One-page profile

This describes what is important to the person and how to support them. It will show us the areas of the person's life where they want to make decisions.

Communication chart

This helps us to understand how the person communicates, particularly if they do not use many words. It tells us what the person's behaviour is telling us and what we need to do.

Person-centred reviews

A way for the person and their family to reflect on their life and services, and look at what is working and not working, and setting actions for change.

One-page profile

This tells us in detail how the person wants to live each day, and what needs to happen to support them well. This is a 'job description' for staff, about what personalisation means for that individual.

Decision-making agreement

This identifies the decisions that the person makes or wants to make and how staff need to support them.

Working Together for Change

This is a way to take information from person-centred reviews to inform how services and organisations need to change.

" I have personal choice and control or influence over decisions about me "

" I know that services are designed around me and my needs "

" I have support that helps me live my life "

National Dementia Declaration - What people affected by dementia have said they want to see in their lives

One-page profile

We need to know what good support looks like for people and this is recorded on a one-page profile.

" I have a sense of belonging and of being a valued part of family, community and civic life "

What people affected by dementia have said they want to see in their lives and how person-centred practices can help

Relationship circles

Helps us understand who is in the person's life and how these relationships can be supported.

Community map

The places where the person goes to in their community.

Presence to contribution

A way to look at how to support the person to go from being present in their community, to having a valued role and making a contribution.

Figure 2.2 How person-centred practices help deliver what people with dementia want

Each person-centred thinking tool does two things. It is the basis for actions and it provides further information about what is important to the person and how she wants to be supported. This information is recorded as a person-centred description and may start with information on just one page (a 'one-page profile'). In the rest of this book we will explore a range of person-centred thinking tools and practices. At the end, you should be familiar with and have read examples and stories about one-page profiles, relationship circles, communication charts, decision-making agreements, working and not working from difference perspectives, person-centred reviews, 'if I could I would…', community maps, and presence to contribution. We start with the key to the first stage of delivering personalisation to people living with dementia: one-page profiles.

Chapter 3
Knowing the Person

One-Page Profiles

It is in the fine grain of care that quality care is really experienced, the tiny details that show that our uniqueness has been recognised.

Mary Marshall in the preface to Living Fuller Lives (2007)

Just because people have dementia this doesn't mean that they don't know what they want.

Sally Percival, Carer and Chair of the National Co-Production Group

If people would ask me I can still tell them what I want, I just need a bit more help getting those things these days. I can't just go and have a coffee in my favourite café because I may not find my way back. Life isn't worth living without those small joys so what do we do?

Louisa, who is living with dementia

Personalisation starts with the person: knowing who they are, what matters to them and how they want to be supported. A *one-page profile* therefore is the foundation of personalisation. Without this information, people are likely to be treated as a clinical condition – and their dementia will always be seen first.

A one-page profile describes what people value about someone, what is individual about them, what is important to them and how best to support them. It reflects the balance between what is important to the person and how we can ensure they stay as healthy, safe and well as possible. Doreen is 84 and lives in a care home. Figure 3.1 shows Doreen's one-page profile.

Doreen's one-page profile

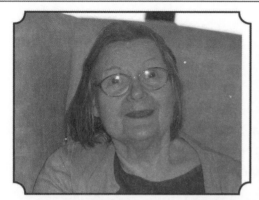

What people appreciate about Doreen

- A good solid woman, you would always want her in your corner.
- Her easy, gentle way with everyone ('kings and mice alike').
- She is full of joy and life.
- Her integrity – she restores your faith in human nature.
- A real people person – friendly and warm.

What is important to Doreen

- Seeing and making other people happy.
- Clifford her husband and Janet her daughter whom she sees every week.
- Seeing her son Keith, who lives in Bristol, as often as possible.
- Her grandchildren Caroline, Gareth, Emma, Andrew and Edward – she is very proud of all of her grandchildren.
- Reading the newspaper each day – The Daily Express.
- Sitting outside in the garden when the weather is fine or looking out of the window at the trees.
- Baking whenever she can.
- Singing – Doreen can often be heard humming a tune or singing aloud (she will tell you she knows all the words and her favourite depends on her mood on the day!). The 50s, 60s and 70s tunes are her favourites.
- Knitting.
- Getting out to Stockport to watch the old shows at The Plaza or having afternoon tea there.
- Celebrating her birthday each year with the people she shares her home with, and with the entertainers and cakes that Clifford brings in for everybody.
- Having Christmas dinner each year at The Midway and seeing all the Christmas celebrations – it has always been her favourite time of year.
- Going out for a pub lunch whenever she can.
- Never to be ignored.
- A varied routine, for example events at the home such as car boot sales, barbeques – anything different to the usual routine which brings people together.
- Being around people and having a good chat, especially with Winifred and Kathleen.
- Getting away for a weekend break occasionally.
- Going to church (St Paul's) on Sundays, especially the 11.00am service.

How best to support Doreen

- It works better for Doreen to go out in the afternoon rather than later in the evening.
- Doreen needs to use a wheelchair if she is outdoors.
- Doreen gets up in her own time between 8.00am and 10.00am each morning.
- Doreen will tell people if she is becoming frustrated and wants her own space – support her to find a quiet corner or to go to her room.
- Doreen should be supported to sleep on her side each night and a pillow positioned behind her so as she doesn't roll onto her back. She needs to be facing the side of the bed she gets out on so she is able to get up when she is ready without needing support.
- If Doreen has back pain, she may want to have breakfast in her bedroom.

Figure 3.1 Doreen's one-page profile

If your first contact with Doreen was reading her care plan, then Figure 3.2 shows how she is described.

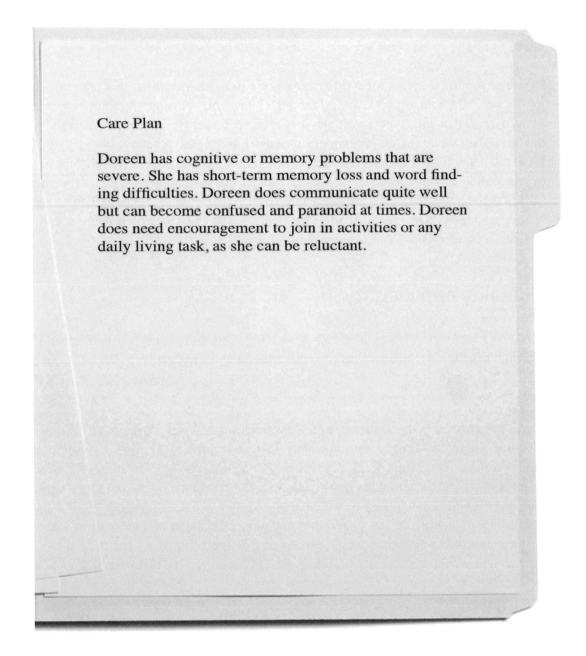

Care Plan

Doreen has cognitive or memory problems that are severe. She has short-term memory loss and word finding difficulties. Doreen does communicate quite well but can become confused and paranoid at times. Doreen does need encouragement to join in activities or any daily living task, as she can be reluctant.

Figure 3.2 Extract from Doreen's care plan

Obviously, you get a very different understanding of who Doreen is from her one-page profile compared with her care plan. Many organisations put a lot of effort into their care plans and they can contain good person-centred information, similar to some of the information about Doreen in her one-page profile. Even in the best care plans we have seen, however, crucial information about the person can be scattered across 60 pages of mainly clinical information and assessments, or be a page of 'likes and dislikes', with a life story. Many care homes are good at recording a person's life story with them. Life stories are important and can provide direct information or clues about what matters to the person now, but doing a life story does not replace detailed knowledge of what is important to someone *now*. If someone has been a vegetarian for their whole life, this does not necessarily mean that they no longer want to eat meat.

Ken Clasper spoke about living well with dementia at the Tyne and Wear Care Alliance Dementia Conference in Gateshead in November 2012. He talked about how drastically his tastes have changed since his diagnosis of Lewy Body dementia – for instance, his preferences concerning food and music. This stresses the importance of living stories – past, present and future.

You rarely read in care plans the positive, valued characteristics of the person, the rich detail of who they are – their important relationships and connections, passions, hobbies and interests – in so much detail that you know which newspaper matters, or what their culture or faith means to them, other than a tick box on admission about which religion they follow.

This depth of knowledge about what is important to someone is central to person-centred care and personalisation, as Dawn Brooker (2007) says in her definition of person-centred dementia care: 'Treating people as individuals; appreciating that all people with dementia have a unique history and personality, physical and mental health, and social and economic resources, and that these will affect their response to neurological impairment.'

Individuality and identity

High quality care is synonymous with respecting individuality.

Gibson 2004, p.55

Individuality is reflected in the well-respected VIPS framework, where the 'I' in VIPS stands for 'An Individual Approach, recognising uniqueness' (Brooker 2007, p.13). One of the indicators Dawn Brooker looks for through VIPS is Individual Preferences, asking: 'Are individual likes and dislikes, preferences and daily routines known about by direct care staff and acted upon?' (p.133).

A one-page profile is a summary of what matters to someone now and goes beyond simple likes and dislikes to identify the key preferences and unique attributes that make them who they are. The profile records what other people like, admire or appreciate about the individual. This reflects a move in the direction of what Bartlett and O'Connor (2010, p.41) describe as moving from 'personhood' to 'citizenship'. They encourage us to go further than identity and think about social positions and roles. Doreen's one-page profile reflects her social positions and roles as wife, mother and grandmother. Early thinking about personhood assumed that people with dementia experienced a loss of self. This view has been challenged and now loss of identity is seen as a potential hazard rather than inevitable. Now we are more concerned with ways to maintain identity, and a one-page profile can contribute to this.

The third section of a one-page page profile is a summary of the key information needed to keep the person healthy, safe and well. This differs from typical clinical information in two ways:

1. It describes how the person wants to be supported. For example, Doreen's one-page profile tells us that she gets up in her own time, between 8am and 10am in the morning.

2. It reflects the balance that we need to achieve between what is important *to* the person, and what matters *for* them to stay healthy, safe and well.

Getting a balance between what is important *to* and *for* a person

The National Dementia Declaration emphasises the importance of supporting people living with dementia in ways that makes sense to them (statement 3 of the Declaration).

In a one-page profile the 'how best to support me' section contributes to the job description for everyone supporting the person.

A one-page profile reflects what we have learned about what matters to the person, and the best ways to support people, to help them stay healthy, safe and well, in the way that makes sense to them (Sanderson and Lewis 2012). The idea of the balance between what is *important to* and what is *important for* a person is rooted in the human condition where none of us has a life where we have everything that is *important to* us and none of us pays perfect attention to everything that is *important for* us. All of us strive for a balance between them that acknowledges issues of health and well-being but recognises that perfect well-being is rarely achieved, while all of us address what is *important for* us in the context of what is *important to* us. This is a human issue, not just a disability issue (Michael Smull, in Sanderson and Lewis 2012). This is the first and fundamental person-centred thinking skill – the ability to learn what is important to someone, what is important for her and the balance between the two.

Historically, people living with dementia have been subjected to the effects of what Kitwood (1997) calls Malignant Social Psychology (MSP). A person's identity is undermined by MSP by treating people as if they were children (infantilisation), by negatively labelling and stereotyping people, and being disparaging about them. Positive Person Work (PPW) emphasises identity through respecting the person, accepting them and celebrating achievements. In person-centred practices, this is extended to ensure that what matters to the person is present in their life and that they are supported in the way that they want to be.

As Michael Smull says, learning what is *important to* and what is *important for* has to be done before you can help find the balance (Sanderson and Lewis 2012). Everyone finds that what is important *to* them and what is important *for* them are in conflict from time to time. For instance, most of us try to find a balance between eating healthy and unhealthy food and drink, to keep our weight stable and enjoy alcohol in moderation. Parents negotiate this balance with or for their children. What is important *to* a person is what she says through her own words and behaviours about what really matters to her. What is important *for* people is what helps them become or stay healthy and safe, whether it is important *to* them or not. Every way that we support someone living with dementia has to take into account what is important to the person now and balancing this with what matters for the person, within the context of the deprivation of liberty safeguards and the Mental Capacity Act 2005.

Here are some examples of what a balance between *important to* and *important for* looks like for five people who are living with dementia:

- It is important to Frank to go out every day, by himself. It is important for Frank to be safe from the traffic on the busy road. The balance between important to and for Frank is for him to be able to go into the grounds of the care home every day, when he chooses, but that the gates remain closed so that he is not able to get on to the main road.

- It is important to Audrey to eat only bananas and nothing else. It is important for her to have a balanced diet, so the staff supporting Audrey have achieved the balance by giving her food supplement drinks.

- It is important to Grace that she walks independently whenever possible and does not use a walking frame. It is important for Grace to be safe from falls, so staff encourage her to use her frame in the dining room where it is busy, but not in her own room.

- It is important to Edie to go home. She wants to return to her family home at night, to be with her mum. Her mum died years ago and there is no family home now, so it is important for Edie not to leave the care home at night to try to get home. The balance for Edie is for staff to talk gently to her about it being too dark to leave in the evening, and to stay.

- It is important to June to have her walking frame with her at all times and never for it to be out of range for her. It is important for June to sleep, but she cannot sleep without having her walking frame in her hand. The balance for June is for her to have her frame on her bed so that she can sleep as close to it as possible.

To find the balance between what matters to the person and staying safe and well, we need to know:

- What is important to a person?

- What is important for a person?

- What else do we need to learn?

These three questions look deceptively simple, but experience tells us that asking these directly rarely works. Seeing a one-page profile as a new form to fill out and just asking people or their relatives 'What is important to you?' and 'How do you want to be supported?' is unlikely to lead to the rich information that we need. This information is drawn out through conversation, learning about people in different ways, and a one-page profile is simply a way to structure how we record this information. We learn about people and discover this information by asking about morning routines, good days and bad days, and by listening to the expertise and learning of family and staff. In the rest of this chapter we look at these person-centred thinking tools and show how to gather this information and record it in a one-page profile (Figure 3.3).

One-page profile

Photo

Each one-page profile has a current photo of the person.

Appreciations

This section summarises the person's positive characteristics, qualities and talents. It can also be called 'like and admire'. It is not a list of accomplishments or awards, but it reflects what others value and appreciate about the person. It needs to have strong, positive statements, and not 'usually' or 'sometimes'.

What is important to the person

This is a bullet list of what really matters to the person from their perspective (even if others do not agree). It is detailed and specific. This section needs to have enough detail so that someone who does not know the person can understand who they are. It is not a list of likes and dislikes, but it reflects what and who is most important to the person.

The detail is crucial. It should not be a list of two-word bullet points like 'having fun', but should instead provide a detailed explanation of what that means to the person - for example: '(Name) enjoys harmless practical jokes and time to sit and relax with people over lunch or coffee.' It should not include 'regularly' as this means different things to different people; instead, say specifically how often – daily? weekly? monthly? Rather than saying 'friends' or 'family', write people's names.

It could include:
· who the important people are in the person's life, and when and how they spend time together
· important interests and hobbies, and when, where and how often these take place
· possessions that are important to the person
· information about the rhythm and pace of life, and any important routines.

How best to support the person

This is a bullet list of how to support the person and what people need to know or do. It is not a list of general hints, but it is specific enough to enable anyone to support the person and know the most important things to do. It can include both what is helpful and what is not.

Again, the detail is important, so that people would know exactly what good support looks like. For instance, instead of saying 'stay positive', it is more helpful to explain what that means to the person - for example: '(Name) is a glass half-full person and it helps her enormously when people look for solutions and not problems. She finds it very draining if she is the only optimist.'

Figure 3.3 Good practice for one-page profiles

Learning from life stories

Understanding someone's history or life story is a very important way to learn about them, and most care homes pay attention to this, either through a page in the person's care plan or more sophisticated memory boxes, books or film. We explore this in more detail in Chapter 8, but in this section we focus on how you can learn from someone's life story about what matters to them and how to support them well. Individuals' personal backgrounds can help us understand who they are and interpret behaviours that might otherwise be difficult to understand, particularly when people are unhappy or distressed. People with advanced dementia have lost their ability to lay down new memory for faces and places, and use their old memory to interpret the environment (Milwain 2010). Memories of childhood and early adulthood are often very strong for people with dementia and new memories are integrated into these.

Specific activities in the care home or the particular approach of a member of staff may trigger powerful feelings related to painful events in someone's past. People may have repetitive behaviours and mannerisms that are hard to fathom and there are often clues in people's life stories that can help to provide explanations and can therefore inform you how best to support the person.

Here are some examples:

- Marion had been a health visitor for most of her working life. She regularly became distressed in a home where dolls were used because people were carrying them by their hair and she was concerned about this abuse of the 'babies'. The best way to support Marion was for her to sit with Ethel who cherished the doll/baby, which she often sat and held. We also asked Marion to fill out the daily records – she would sit and record her visits over the years into a log book and it appeared to give her a valued role, which she took great pride in.

- Betty would go rigid when the ironing board came out – her husband used to burn her with the iron. In Betty's one-page profile, in the support section it says: 'Never iron where Betty can see you. If she does see the iron, sit with her, comfort her, stroking her hand and letting her know she is OK and you are OK.'

- Pauline would cry out when she saw the hairdresser with the hair rollers – she was assaulted and hair rollers pushed into her head caused severe damage to her scalp and skull. Good support for Pauline is always to ensure she is working – folding the laundry or sewing are favourites – well away from the hairdresser's room.

- Joe, a former security guard, would continually check doors. On Joe's one-page profile it says: 'Know that Joe was a security guard for many years and will continually check doors before going to bed. Leave him be; he will be happy to go to bed once he knows he has checked every door. Rushing him will make him anxious and angry.'

As well as beginning to learn how to support people well, life stories also provide information or clues to what and who are still important to the person now. Edie's story shows how life stories are an important way to get to know someone, but that what was important in the past may no longer be important now. Edie is a well-known character locally, renowned for her straight talking and described as the 'salt of the earth'. She lives in a care home. Here is part of her life story.

Information from Edie's life story

- Baking – Edie always loved to bake.

- A keen knitter. Also, Edie spent many happy hours crocheting.

- She loved to walk and would walk for miles.

- Visiting Stockport market each week was a must!

- Watching Victor Mature films.

- Edie's favourite pastime was reading. She was always buying books – Catherine Cookson was her favourite author.

Figure 3.4 shows how what was important to Edie in the past has either changed or is still reflected in what is important to her now.

Important to Edie in the past	What is important to Edie now
• Baking – Edie always loved to bake.	• Edie's well-being is clearly increased when she sits near the kitchen hatch and watches the cook baking cakes. She has commented several times, 'It smells just like my Mam's kitchen'.
• A keen knitter. Edie also spent many happy hours crocheting.	• Edie has threatened people with the knitting needles and she has no interest in knitting any more.
• She loved to walk and would walk for miles.	• We have tried going out with Edie several times but on each occasion she has cried out 'kidnap'. We know she loves to feel the wind and smell fresh air so she spends a large part of the day and evening sitting by the front doors in one of the easy chairs or in the garden if it's warm.
• Visiting Stockport market each week.	• Edie loves to set out tables in the home as though market stalls and is animated when rummaging through the goods.
• Watching Victor Mature films like 'My Darling Clemintine'.	• Edie is no longer interested in watching films.
• Edie's favourite pastime was reading. She was always buying books – Catherine Cookson was her favourite author.	• Edie can no longer read.

Figure 3.4 What was important to Edie in the past and now

Learning about good days and bad days

Good days and bad days is a person-centred thinking tool that simply asks the person to describe what a typical day is like, starting with when she wakes up and continuing until she goes to bed. Then you can ask for the same detailed information about what an especially good day is like and a particularly bad day. This tells you what needs to be present for her in her day-to-day life and what needs to be absent, and both would be recorded as what is important to the person.

For Doreen, it's a good day when she been talking to Winifred and Kathleen, and a bad day when she's been ignored. Both appear in 'what is important to Doreen' in her one-page profile.

In reality, the conversation is likely to meander. Some people cannot describe a good day or a bad day, but they can tell you about the last week in great detail, so that you can gently ask which bits of the day were good and which not so good. If the person has not had good days for some time, she may be able to tell you about a good day from her past.

When the person cannot tell you directly herself, then family or support staff can help. You could ask: 'If you had a magic wand and were going to create a really good day for the person, what would happen? What would she be doing? Who else would be there?' And then ask a similar question about a bad day: 'What would you do if you wanted to ruin someone's day?' This teases out both what matters to the person (what is important) and what needs to happen for them to have a good day or avoid a bad day (this often gives us information about how to support the person well).

As well as being an important person-centred thinking tool for learning about what is important to someone and how to support them, you can use this information to start to improve the person's life immediately, by asking, 'What would it take for you to have more good days and fewer bad days?'

Louisa's good and bad days

Louisa is a fun-loving, sociable 70-year-old who is described as so generous she would give you her last penny. She has recently been diagnosed with Lewy Body dementia. She lives in her own home, which she shared with her husband Bill for many years until his death a year ago. Louisa cared for Bill, who had motor neurone disease. A very independent woman, Louisa was a head teacher in a secondary school until her retirement nine years ago. Her memory has become increasingly impaired, so her son and daughter call regularly to support her to remain at home. This is supplemented with calls four times each day from a homecare service.

Louisa goes through phases of really struggling to swallow; investigations have not revealed any medical reason and anxiety is suspected at this point. Her family are concerned about Louisa's sleeping as she is afraid to go upstairs to bed and has been using the recliner chair as her bed downstairs.

Louisa and her Admiral nurse, Bernie, used the *good days and bad days* tool to have conversations about what it would take for Louisa to have more good days. Here is Louisa's good days and bad days information (Figure 3.5).

Good day	Bad day
• Staff are on time so I can have my breakfast before 9.30am.	• A carer I do not know turns up at my door, especially bad if I haven't been forewarned.
• Dial-a-Ride come on time so I have a nice lunch with friends at the luncheon club.	• I feel a burden on Joanne and Michael.
• Hearing from Vi and planning a visit.	• Everybody is telling me to sleep in the bed and I detest going upstairs.
• Sunday roast with my family.	• Joanne is stressed and upset when she visits and I do not know what I have done or what has happened to distress her. She says everything is fine but I wonder if I got lost and have forgotten.
• My stamina is good and I am thinking well.	
• Sue or Theresa are the carers who call.	
• Joanne, my daughter, or Michael, my son, visit.	• I wake from bad nightmares.
• I can wash myself before the carers arrive in the morning.	• I go out and do not know how to get home – this is my worst nightmare.
• I have a real sense of who I am and 'feel on form'.	• I feel as though I have no hope and my future is one where I know I am in a bad situation but have no concept that I have dementia.
• I don't need to look at the instructions Joanne has left to do the tasks which have been so familiar to me such as making a drink.	
• I can multi-task as I always did without any confusion.	• I need to sleep most of the day.
	• I go to get in my car and realise I am no longer allowed to drive.
• I wake refreshed after a comfy night on my recliner chair.	• I feel my life is in everybody else's hands and I have no control.
• I make a nice meal for Joanne and Michael to come and share with me.	• I have the shakes badly.
• Going to church and seeing friends there	• I feel undignified when my swallow is poor and I spill my drink down me.
• Watching comedies on the TV.	• I believe people are stealing my things, especially when carers I don't know turn up.
• There are fresh flowers in the house.	
• Having a call or seeing an ex-pupil.	• I am anxious and can't put my finger on why.
	• I answer the telephone but have no idea whose voice it is although they obviously know me well.
	• Not having a newspaper to read.

Figure 3.5 Louisa's good days and bad days

Her good days include seeing friends at the luncheon club, her family and the carers she knows well, suggesting that those things are very important to her. On her bad days she feels reliant on others and that her life is in the hands of others, suggesting that to support her well is to help her do things rather than taking over and leaving her feeling disempowered.

Bernie and Louisa used this information to build her one-page profile and also began to think together about the decisions Louisa was keen to make for herself. We explain in more detail about one-page profiles and decision making later in the book (see Chapter 4).

What do Louisa's good days and bad days tell us about what is important to her and how to support her well? Figure 3.5 shows what her first draft one-page profile looked like.

Louisa's one-page profile

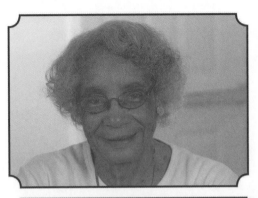

What is important to Louisa

- Her daughter Joanne and son Michael.
- Ethel, Vi, Edith and Jim, friends Louisa sees every week at luncheon club.
- Visiting Marie her niece who lives in Devon, going to stay with her for a week each summer.
- Going about her daily business – cleaning the house, going to the shops without feeling confused, tired or overwhelmed.
- To have something to offer such as cooking a Sunday roast for Joanne and Michael to enjoy with her.
- Comedies on the TV and having a good old laugh – 'You can't beat it, I love to laugh.'
- Good conversation.
- To continue to live well and do the things she did prior to her diagnosis of dementia
- Being ready for the day after a good sleep and breakfast – not waiting around for the home care service.
- That Sue or Theresa provide her support.
- To go to church, see friends there, especially Audrey and Sheila, having a coffee with friends in the church hall after the service.
- Having a daily newspaper to read – *The Daily Express* is her favourite.
- Having coffee during the day and a cup of tea at teatime. Horlicks in the evening is a must!
- Fresh flowers – Louisa loves them!
- Old friends from school (where Louisa was the head) and ex-pupils visiting.
- Having a heart to heart with Bernie, the Admiral Nurse – 'You can't beat it; Bernie gives me so much strength and belief that I can live well with dementia.'

What people appreciate about Louisa

- Very determined.
- Generous.
- Loving.
- A caring Mum.

How best to support Louisa

- Louisa's day will be ruined if she is not organised for the day by 9.30am; therefore her breakfast call needs to be before 9.00am.
- Louisa will tell you that she tends to get lost when outdoors and she finds this terrifying and humiliating. Be sensitive – she appreciates others being aware of this and encouragement to stay strong. She welcomes any offers to accompany her outdoors, especially to the Trafford Centre; for example to have a shopping trip together.
- Louisa has days when she is incredibly tired and cannot think straight. She will become very distressed, so sitting talking to her and reassuring her that there are people around her to help will offer her comfort. Watching a comedy or going out for a drive (over Woodhead preferably) will often lift her mood.
- If a carer Louisa does not know is having to provide support, always telephone her in advance to forewarn her.
- Do not 'do for' Louisa. She wants to be part of a team taking as much control as she can – with you, working together.
- Louisa sleeps on her recliner chair. Do not nag her to use the bed, she has a real fear of being upstairs alone.
- Be honest with Louisa. She will worry more if she senses something is wrong but you are keeping it from her.
- If Louisa is shaking and asks you to help her with it, be aware she has some PRN meds – see care plan for detail.
- Be aware that if Louisa is struggling to swallow, she uses a beaker with a lid and blends her food. Do not interfere with this as Louisa feels strongly these decisions are down to her with advice from the dietician and GP.
- When telephoning Louisa, always say who it is when she answers.

Figure 3.6 Louisa's one-page profile

As a result of doing *good days and bad days*, Louisa both had a one-page profile to share with her family and workers, and she and Bernie made the following changes to help her have more good days:

1. Sue and Theresa are now Louisa's named workers from the agency providing support.

2. The contract stipulates Louisa's morning call must happen between 8am and 8.45am.

3. Louisa is looking at getting an electronic bed for the front room with the help of an occupational therapist who has been referred to support Louisa with this.

May's good days and bad days

May also used the *good days and bad days* person-centred thinking tool with Paula, her key worker, at the care home where she lives (Figure 3.7). If you met May, she would probably enjoy telling you about her years as an advertising executive and the 'huge ghastly advertising boards' she had put up around Stockport. She would also tell you wonderful stories of the time she spent as commissioner of all the Guide troops in South Stockport.

May has lived at Bruce Lodge since June 2010 and is in the early- to middle-stage experience of her dementia. May and Paula thought about what made a good day and those things that would be happening if it was a bad day. Paula used this to frame their conversation in order to develop her one-page profile.

Looking at May's good days and bad days provides rich, detailed information about what is important to her, and clues about what support she wants and needs. Like Louisa, it is also a way to have conversations that lead to action so that the people supporting her can help her have more good days than bad. So we begin to inform the one-page profiles from these conversations knowing what matters to May, which things increase her well-being and how best to support her.

The big outcome for May from her good days and bad days was creating a one-page profile where the 'how best to support her' then became part of the job description. This helps staff to ensure these things are present on a day-to-day basis and that she is consistently supported in a way that makes sense to her even if there are lots of different staff involved in her support.

Using the *good days and bad days* tool is the first step towards making a person's day-to-day experience how they want it to be. Paula started to learn about May differently through looking at her good days and bad days, and then went on to learn about routines as well. From both of these, she began May's one-page profile with her.

<table>
<tr><td>

Good day

- Time to relax with a glass of wine and a good book.
- Going to mass and taking communion at St Joseph's Church.
- Going to the coffee mornings or other events at Our Lady of the Apostles Church.
- Marie visits me, or other friends from church come over.
- Having a day out with Marie.
- Seeing Janice who was in my Brownie troop.
- Chatting with other people who live here and talking 'good sense'.
- Having a good night's sleep without worrying or becoming anxious about what is going on and why I live here, followed by enjoying my breakfast in peace.
- I know what day it is and the date; 'in fact the days when I'm with it and can remember things I have done in my life.'
- Getting outdoors to do different things – 'I don't mind what – just a change of scenery, I do like a good old rummage in the markets, though.'

</td><td>

Bad day

- People are quizzing me for no good reason.
- I can't work out why I live here with these other people.
- I don't know the day or date; 'that really gets me worked up, it's terrible you know when you can't remember things.'
- Thinking I'm in a mess because I don't know what's going on or why I am living here.
- I'm not sure if my brother Anthony and sister Bridget are still alive – then realise they are dead.
- I can't recall if I still see Janice, my friend, or my niece, Marie.
- No newspaper to read; last week's is no good to me at all!
- Not to go to mass.

</td></tr>
</table>

Figure 3.7 May's good days and bad days

Learning about important routines

Routines are a way to ease ourselves through the day. Finding out about someone's routines is a great way to learn about what matters and what support the person needs.

Here are some routines to have conversations about:

- What is your *morning routine*? How do you wake up in the morning? What happens next? Tell me about breakfast.

- What is your *evening routine*? What do you do to get ready for bed? What do you do next?

- *Routines for comfort.* What do you do when you have had a bad day? How do you try and cheer yourself up?

- *Routines for celebration.* What is your favourite way to celebrate? What would you do after a particularly good day? What would you do to celebrate good news or achievements? How do you like to celebrate your birthday? What else would you always celebrate? What religious or cultural festivals do you celebrate? How do you celebrate?

- *Transition routines.* What do you do when you first get to work or the day centre? What do you do as soon as you get home?

- *Weekly routines.* What do you do almost without fail every week? Are there any TV programmes that you just have to see? What are they? Are there people you see every week? What else do you do each week?

May's routines are central to her well-being – any move away from them can leave her disorientated and distressed. Figure 3.8 describes May's morning routine.

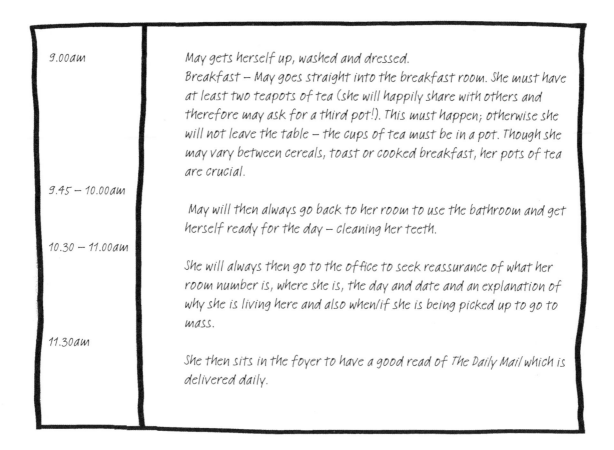

9.00am	May gets herself up, washed and dressed. Breakfast – May goes straight into the breakfast room. She must have at least two teapots of tea (she will happily share with others and therefore may ask for a third pot!). This must happen; otherwise she will not leave the table – the cups of tea must be in a pot. Though she may vary between cereals, toast or cooked breakfast, her pots of tea are crucial.
9.45 – 10.00am	May will then always go back to her room to use the bathroom and get herself ready for the day – cleaning her teeth.
10.30 – 11.00am	She will always then go to the office to seek reassurance of what her room number is, where she is, the day and date and an explanation of why she is living here and also when/if she is being picked up to go to mass.
11.30am	She then sits in the foyer to have a good read of The Daily Mail which is delivered daily.

Figure 3.8 May's morning routine

May doesn't have specific routines during the day as she will usually 'go with the flow' (in her words) but after tea she always goes up and gets ready for bed and then comes back down in the lift in her dressing gown and asks for her wine glass from the office. This is a cue that she wants a glass of wine or two, but she will tell you it could lead to more – May's view is 'never fly on one wing'. She often then sits in the foyer and reads a novel while drinking her wine. May goes up to bed around 10pm but will always call in the office to collect an empty glass so she can have a glass of water by her bed during the night. There is another routine that is crucial in May's life – she goes to mass on a Sunday.

Paula used what she had learned with May from her *good days and bad days* and her routines to develop her one-page profile (Figure 3.9). Sharing this with staff made a huge difference to how they supported May. Later they used it to find out what was working and not working for May, and to change what was not working for her, and we talk about this later in the book (see Chapter 6).

May's one-page profile

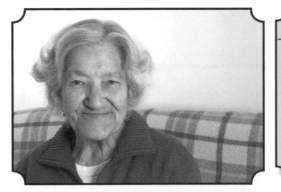

What people appreciate about May

- Gregarious – 'Beaming personality' 'great character'.
- Wicked sense of fun.
- Diplomatic – May has a gift to say it as it is without ever being rude.
- Refined – with beautiful manners.
- Helpful.

What is important to May

- Her niece Marie; going out together and going on holiday together.
- Pots of tea each morning at breakfast (at least two to share).
- To know what the date is.
- Her friend Sharon and other friends from church, and Janice who was in May's Brownie troop.
- May must go to weekday and Sunday masses (St Joseph's in Stockport) and take communion at church.
- To go to the coffee mornings and social events at Our Lady of the Apostles on Shaw Heath.
- To talk about her late sister Bridget who was a supervisor of nursing.
- Being around others and having a good chat.
- Having a purpose in her day and helping other people.
- Talking about her life – about her years as an advertising executive and the 'huge ghastly advertising boards' she had put up around Stockport.
- Not to be 'queried' by staff.
- A glass or two of dry white wine each evening.
- A gin and tonic now and again, 'for a change is good'.
- Spending time chatting with Margaret, Mary A, Blanche and Doreen who live here.
- Going 'out and about' whenever she can; for example, to the market.

How best to support May

- Remind May often of the date.
- May will often ask how long she has lived here (she moved in June 2010) and why she lives here: 'Is it a place for crackpot old people?' Reassure her this is not the case and that she's here so that she has people around to help her; for example, looking after her laundry, cleaning, cooking and generally there is always someone to turn to if she needs any help.
- Always explain to May why you need any information from her (so she does not feel 'queried').
- Show May the way to Fern Lounge frequently where she enjoys the company and conversation of her particular group of friends who live here.
- Know that on the record May is named as Mary Francis. This would be important if she was ever going to hospital; for example, where you should tell hospital staff that she is known as May.

Figure 3.9 May's one-page profile

Learning from family and staff

Family members are a mine of rich information about their loved one and it is vital that they are involved in sharing this. An easy way to do this is to ask them, and other people who know the person well, for their 'top tips' for providing great support. Here is a useful question to ask: 'If you had only two minutes to share your top tips about supporting (name of individual) well, what would you say?'

John, Ann's husband, helped staff learn about Ann using this approach. Ann lives in a residential home for people with dementia. She was not able to talk much about her routines or her good days and bad days, and staff learned more about her from John. Joanne, Ann's key worker, asked John for his top tips for supporting Ann. This is what he said:

> First and foremost if Ann does not want to do something no amount of persuasion will change her mind. Although Ann enjoys helping others she will let them know when she's had enough of them. Never leave her alone with anybody who makes a lot of noise because that will push her to the point of hitting out, as she is unable to think through that walking away is a better option.
>
> Ann reacts best if you explain clearly what you would like her to do – preferably by showing her.
>
> Never try to get her hair cut!
>
> Little things cheer Ann like a conversation about a lovely picture on the wall.
>
> Her frame of mind can change very quickly.
>
> If Ann doesn't like the look of what is in front of her, no amount of encouragement would sway her to eat it – it would only distress her so leave it.
>
> Ann becomes incredibly upset about her personal care, you would need to know her well before supporting her with this.
>
> If Ann tells you to 'bugger off', leave her be.
>
> I must always be present if Ann is seeing the GP or podiatrist.
>
> Never hug Ann unless she hugs you.
>
> Going outdoors in the fresh air calms her if she is in a state of ill-being.

If you can understand who Ann likes to be with, and equally the people she does not like to be with, then you are halfway there. Also, when Ann gets anxious or does not want to do something, leave it and try again later, as Ann's mood does change very quickly. She needs to clearly understand what you are going to do if you are helping her in any way and showing her first works best.

This gives lots of information about what is important to Ann and what is important for her so that people can support her well.

What this tells us about how to support Ann

- Although Ann enjoys helping others, pay attention to the fact that she will let them know when she has had enough of them.

- If you are new, watch and learn from other people who know Ann well before supporting her. She becomes incredibly upset about her personal care and you would need to know her well before supporting her with this.

- Know that Ann's frame of mind can change very quickly.

- Ann only has her hair cut when necessary – she detests it and would only ever be supported by John when having it done.

- John must always be present if Ann is seeing the GP or podiatrist.

It's vital to work proactively with family members and ensure we capture their important contribution.

Learning about important people – relationship circles

What is important to someone will almost always include people – family, friends, neighbours, colleagues. Mike Nolan, in his 'relationship-centred care', emphasises the importance of people having a sense of belonging and 'opportunities to maintain and/or create meaningful and reciprocal relationships. To feel part of a community or group as desired' (Nolan 2004, p.50).

We can learn about and record the important people in someone's life by having conversations and using the person-centred thinking tool call the *relationship circle*. This is the start of thinking about ways to deepen or create opportunities for relationships.

A relationship circle is particularly useful for exploring:

- Who a person knows.

- How they know them.

- Who knows whom.

- How these networks can help the person find opportunities and support to live the life they want.

- Who gets on best with the person and what this means for getting the best staff or volunteer 'match'.

These relationships can be represented as a circle, in columns or as a spider diagram with the person at the centre. In whatever way it is represented, it is vital to be clear not just about who is in the person's life, but how important they are to them. Typically, this is done by putting the person's name or photo in the middle and the names of the people who are most important in her life closest to her.

If you are doing this using the rings of a relationship circle, then the people in the closest ring would be people the person loves; the second ring would be people the person likes; the third ring would be people the person knows; and the final ring would be people who are paid to be in that person's life, such as support staff, hairdressers or GPs.

This process not only identifies who is important in the person's life but can suggest how they can stay in contact and whether any support is needed to keep and develop those relationships. If people find that their relationship circle is not as full as they would like, then it can be become a focus for action by asking: 'What would it take to increase the number and depth of someone's relationships?'

What we appreciate about someone is also crucial for developing and building a relationship with them, so for staff it is a critical but often overlooked first step in getting to know someone.

Olive moved into a residential service supporting people living with dementia six months ago. The homecare service felt it was no longer possible for them to support her within the extra care housing scheme that had been her home for the previous 15 years. Olive's son, Brian, found that thinking about what he appreciated about Olive helped him rediscover his relationship with her. This is how he described her:

> Mum has an impish and very sharp sense of humour. I have a fridge magnet present from her with the slogan 'Don't trust a doctor whose house plants are always dead!' I am a doctor of horticulture!
>
> An excellent knitter, with the ability to adapt patterns to fit us long-armed men!
>
> She played the piano well. I particularly remember her playing *Für Elise*.
>
> She was an awesome bargain hunter!
>
> I remember her telling us how she won a beauty contest in her teens.
>
> Mum was a meticulous painter. I remember the dining room window ledge being painted with Brolac so you could not see a brush stroke.
>
> Mum is a bit of a perfectionist, which showed in the precise way she used to wrap presents so you could not see the paper join.

Brian felt that it was important for his mum to stay connected with family and friends, and also that staff supporting her were able to chat with her about the people in her life, given that Olive had always been such a 'people person'. He completed a relationship circle that identified all the people in Olive's life and the range of different relationships she had with others (Figure 3.10). Brian felt that understanding the network of Olive's relationships would help family and friends to continue to be involved in her life by ensuring that those providing support were aware of and facilitated these relationships to thrive.

This seemed especially important given the huge change in Olive's home situation and the support she now needed due to the rapid progression of her dementia. It also gave a much fuller picture of her life as conversations about the many people Olive knew helped paint the picture of who she was and what her life had been like prior to the onset of dementia. The exercise therefore provided an important first step for staff to get to know Olive, who was in her life and the role they played and could play in providing support and/or enabling her to have a good quality of life.

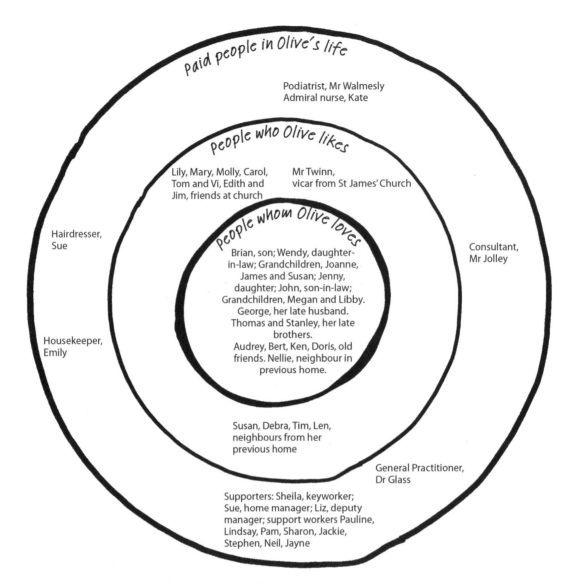

Figure 3.10 Olive's relationship circle

Person-centred thinking tools like *good days and bad days*, *top tips* and *relationship circles* help us know what is important to and for a person, and the balance between them, and this information is recorded and summarised on one page or in a more detailed person-centred description (a one-page profile that goes beyond one page!). We are seeing organisations with a one-page profile for each person they support at the front of the person's file – or even framed in their room.

But what if people aren't always able to be heard? What if they don't use words to communicate? The next chapter will describe the importance of enhancing people's voices and will also take us on to the next step of making decisions – with the person living with dementia – about actions that are needed to bring more choice and control into that person's life.

Chapter 4
Choice and Control in Practice

I may find it hard to say what I mean and come out with muddled words but please continue to listen well to me, stay in touch with me and communicate with me.

Christine Bryden, who was diagnosed with dementia at 46 (Bryden 2012)

If folk would just ask me and give me some time to think it through I would be able to make many more choices than I do right now.

Hazel, who lives in a residential service supporting people living with dementia

I have personal choice and control or influence over decisions about me.

National Dementia Declaration, Dementia Action Alliance

Personalisation requires that we go beyond person-centred care to emphasise supporting people living with dementia to have as much choice and control in their lives as possible. This is central to the National Dementia Declaration and key to the vision for adult health and social care and Think Local, Act Personal. Person-centred thinking tools can help describe how much control people have in their lives by looking at the decisions people can make now. They can also inform what needs to happen to enable people to have more direct control over their lives by increasing the range and depth of the choices they make. This chapter will look at the person-centred thinking tools that enable people to have more choice and control over the decisions being made in their lives.

Having choice, or agency, can in some situations make the difference between life and death. Researchers from Yale and Harvard (Langer 2009) studied nursing home residents to find out what happens when people retain the right to making decisions about their lives and what happens if that right is taken away. They divided residents into two groups of people similar in age, sex and illness. People in the first group were actively encouraged to make decisions about their life in the nursing home, while the others were explicitly encouraged to let staff members make those decisions on their behalf. Everyone was also given a plant for his or her room. Those encouraged to make decisions were given responsibility for keeping the plant alive, while those in the other group were told that staff members would take care of it for them. After 18 months, the researchers analysed the deaths at the nursing home (which had been expected) and found those in the group that couldn't make decisions died at the same rate as was usual for the nursing home, while those in the group that could make decisions died at half the usual rate. The researchers interpreted the findings to mean that those who had more control over decisions in their lives were protected from an earlier death.

For people to have as much choice and control in their lives as possible, we need to know how people communicate (especially if they don't use words) and how people make decisions. This is especially important at the end of their lives. We must also ensure that everyone involved in the person's life has and uses that information. Here are three practical and simple person-centred thinking tools that are good places to start. They can complement the many detailed and sophisticated approaches to communication used by speech and language therapists.

The communication charts

> The world goes much faster than we do, whizzing around, and we are being asked to do things, or respond, or to play a game, or to participate in group activities. If it is too fast, we want to say 'Go away, slow down, leave me alone.' Challenging behaviour? I believe that this is adaptive behaviour where I am adapting to my care environment.
>
> *Christine Bryden (2012)*

The *communication chart* is a powerful way to record how someone communicates. This is a critical tool to have when people do not communicate with words. It is also important to use when people communicate with their behaviour (also known as 'challenging behaviour') or when what people say and what they mean are different, as you can see from Edie's story.

Edie's story

Although Edie uses words, their flow or context can be difficult for us to follow. So if Edie is to have the things that matter to her in her life and as much choice and control as possible, we need to understand what her expressions and words are telling us. For example, once it goes dark in the evening, Edie believes her mum will be worrying about her because she hasn't returned home. Edie will desperately try to leave the home due to her anxiety about her mum; this creates distress for Edie, which gains momentum the longer it goes on.

The team who support Edie have thought about this and their best guess is that Edie is feeling insecure and unloved, seeking the love and security she always found with her mother. Their continual listening and learning has helped them work out that the best way to support Edie is to talk with her about her daughter, Barbara, and reassure her that Barbara will be here in the morning. This works nine times out of ten, though occasionally they have to call Barbara on the telephone so Edie can chat with her. This has been agreed with Barbara and is working well.

Staff supporting Edie have copies of her communication charts so those supporting her can quickly work out what Edie is telling them. Some people carry their communication charts in their bags or keep them in their bedroom to share with staff. As Edie is so fearful of people stealing her things, it works best for staff to have the charts at their fingertips, and this also enables them to add their new learning. This ensures Edie is being heard and that she is consistently supported in a way that makes sense to her, even if there are lots of different staff involved in her support.

Person-centred thinking tools to help with communication

There are the two communication charts that can help us to understand how people 'tell' us what they want and how they make decisions:

- How I communicate with you

- How we communicate with you

The first is a clear, powerful description of how the person communicates (Figure 4.1). In the second, instead of recording what the person does, we record what we are trying to communicate to the person, and then what we are encouraging the person to do (Figure 4.2).

To get started, it is easiest to look at either what the person does or what we think it means, filling in the second or third column first. Start with easy, clear communications such as knowing when the person is angry or sad. How do they demonstrate this? What do you need to do to comfort or support them? How do you know this? When are they most likely to be angry or sad? Getting it started is relatively easy; keeping it alive is the challenge. It needs to be used and revisited on a regular basis. It is crucial to have communication charts in care homes, and families can find it powerful as well, as Joanne did with Doris.

Doris's story

Doris lives at home in Lancashire with her daughter, Joanne, and three teenage granddaughters. Described as a 'real livewire', Doris always has a ready smile and will go out of her way to offer help to others. Joanne thought she was pretty good at best-guessing what many of Doris's behaviours meant – such as the lollipops and taking other people's hats – but she became puzzled by some of the things Doris was doing.

They decided to really pay attention to her life story to see if that might provide clues to explain some of Doris's actions, because as a family they were feeling less and less connected with her. Joanne explained her real fear was that her mum would become isolated in her own bubble and drift further and further away from them unless they learned more about this and were able to step into Mum's reality. Friends and neighbours who had known Doris in her younger years had a crucial part to play in building this portrait of her story. They were able to tell Joanne that Doris had turned to her Roman Catholic faith during the war years and had been a devout worshipper between 1943 and 1949. Joanne was born in 1959 so had never known her mum as a practising Catholic. This helped them work out what some of Doris's actions meant, as described in the communication charts below (Figure 4.3 and 4.4).

Old friends also described how troubled Doris had been about running out of items during rationing. That made Joanne think that her mum's reality right now was those war and post-war years as it explained why Doris was stocking up on so many items. Joanne describes her relief:

We could get closer to Mum simply by stepping into the bubble that is her reality with her and making sure she doesn't drift further and further away from us by being more aware of what she is telling us. There are some things we still don't 'get' but we are constantly trying to learn more rather than just giving up.

At this time	Edie does this	We think it means	And we should
After dark	Says she needs to go as her Mum will be looking for her.	Edie is feeling insecure and unloved.	Talk with Edie, tell her Barbara – her daughter who visits every morning – will be here when it is light. More often than not, this calms Edie, although occasionally you may need to call Barbara so Barbara can reassure her that she will be there in the morning.
Anytime	Grasps her handbag and glares at you.	She does not know or recognise you and is fearful you may snatch her handbag.	Do not approach her – say hello and move on.
In bed	Takes her walking frame into bed and gets comfy under the duvet.	She is fearful somebody will steal her walking frame.	Leave Edie be. She is quite safe and comfortable with the walking frame in the bed.
Anytime	Edie cries 'kidnap'.	She is being asked to do something she doesn't want to do.	Leave Edie be for 10 minutes and then ask again if it is something that needs to happen – her mood does change very quickly.

Figure 4.1 How Edie communicates with us

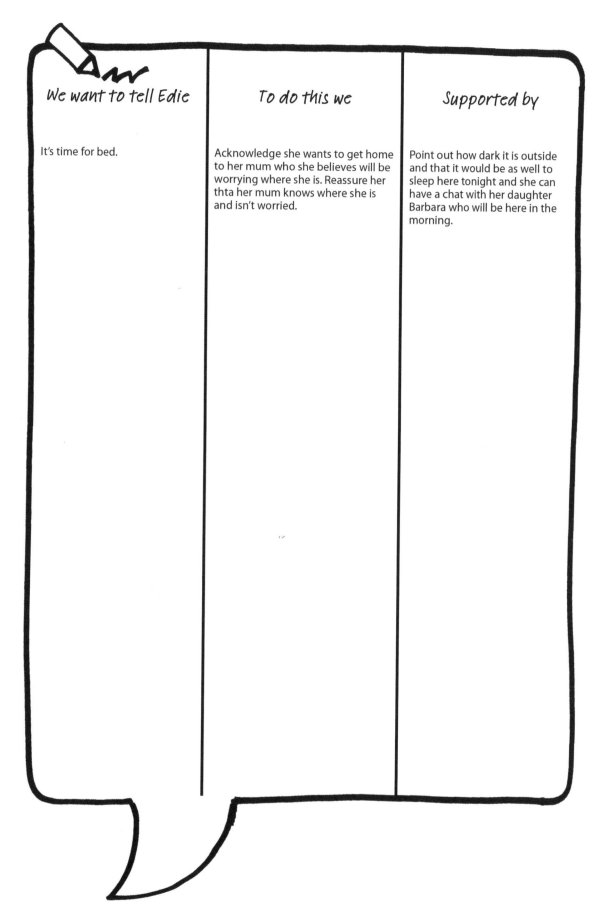

Figure 4.2 How we communicate with Edie

At this time	Doris does this	We think it means	And we should
Anytime	Doris hangs handkerchiefs up around the lounge.	She thinks it is Christmas and is putting decorations up.	Ask what the celebration is, enjoy with her – sit with her and go through her photograph albums which she loves to do.
Anytime	Doris stocks up on items such as A4 batteries, bananas or bathroom cleaner.	She is fearful the shops are running out of stock. Her current reality is the time during the war.	Reassure her we have plenty of food and everything we need in the cupboards.
Anytime	Covers teapot or similar with a handkerchief.	She is thinking of mass and the Eucharist.	Go through the book of minutes she kept from church meetings while listening to her CD of favourite hymns.
Anytime	Lays newspapers or magazines on the breakfast bar and makes a cross on her lips.	She is delivering the gospel reading in church.	Sit quietly with her until she has finished.
Anytime	Doris wants to see what is in the pockets of other people.	She has run out of the lollipops she keeps in her pocket.	Go to the shop with Doris to buy more. If that isn't possible, there is a box in the office. Replenish her supply – 15 will usually last her a week.
When entering a room	Will not move forward to walk in the room.	We are unsure as yet what it means.	Close the door to; Doris will then happily open it and enter the room.
Anytime	Takes hats off other people's heads.	She has run out of hats in her room – Doris always keeps her underwear in a hat before placing it in the drawer.	Go out with her to buy a new hat.

How Doris communicates with us

Figure 4.3 How Doris communicates with us

We want to tell Doris	To do this we	Supported by
It's time for bed.	Ask Doris to turn the TV off.	Offer your arm for Doris to link you and say, 'Shall we go up the dancers.' Never say it's time for bed.

Figure 4.4 How we communicate with Doris

Decision-making agreements

Increasing choice and control of the person's support is at the heart of all personalised service provision.

Think Local, Act Personal

People with dementia have agency. This means the ability to undertake 'actions, activities, decisions and behaviours that represent some measure of meaningful choice'.

Deacon and Mann (1999)

Knowing how someone communicates is essential, yet we need to do more to give people choice and control over their lives. This reflects moving from person-centred care to personalisation. Self-directed support means enabling people to make choices and decisions about how they want to be supported, so that they are in control of the services they receive. There are many studies that demonstrate that people with dementia are able to make decisions and choices, often known as 'agency'. Malcolm Goldsmith emphasises how important it is that staff expect people to make their views and opinions known, even if this is through gestures and non-verbal communication (Goldsmith 1996).

Two areas to think about in decision making are the person's ability to make decisions and who else could or should be involved. A wide range of people may offer formal and informal support – from family and friends, to peers and self-help groups, to faith communities. The full range of people who support someone is not usually identified or acknowledged in the assessment and care planning process, unless a relationship circle is included. Doing a relationship circle (see Chapter 3) is a way for the person to think about and describe those people who are important in his life, and what role they could play in planning and decision making. If there are very few people in the person's life, then the relationship circle could be the beginning of developing goals and outcomes in this area and marking progress. Having important people in your life is not, of course, an automatic passport to shared decision making. Generally, we want to involve different people in different decisions: friends about what to wear for an important event; a partner and family on where to go on holiday; or a business partner on which options to prioritise in the next three months.

People's ability to make decisions is related both to their mental capacity and their opportunities to make decisions. Mental capacity simply means the ability of an individual to make her own decisions, and obviously many people with dementia lack mental capacity. The Mental Capacity Act (2005) established for the first time that people can no longer make decisions on behalf of other people without going through a process. The 'decision-making agreement' is a way to reflect on how decisions are made in the light of this legislation.

The Mental Capacity Act (MCA) and personalisation share core values. The MCA says that a person should make their own decisions and where this is not possible because they lack the mental capacity to do so, that they should play as big a role as possible in decision-making processes that directly affect them. (Social Care Institute of Excellence 2010)

Needing support to make decisions should not prevent people from having control over their lives and exercising their human rights. A decision-making agreement is a way to think about how much control people have over their decisions and how that control can be increased.

A decision-making profile is a person-centred thinking tool that helps staff to know how to support people to make decisions and to reinforce consistency across a team. This delivers more personalised support by working towards increasing the number and significance of the decisions that people make in their lives. When supporting someone in their decision making, here are some important questions to ask:

- Do I fully understand what is important to the person and how they communicate?

- Am I the best person to support this decision making?

- Is the information that I have and am giving the person relevant to the decision?

- Am I presenting it in a way that the person can understand?

- Am I giving the information in the right place and time?

- Have I given the person the best chance to make the decision themselves?

Meg lives in a residential service for people with dementia. The people supporting her wanted to make sure Meg had as much choice and control in her life as possible and so worked with her to develop a *decision-making profile* (Figure 4.5). This person-centred thinking tool shares the person's preferences in the way they want to be supported in decision making.

This information is important to use to assist decision making. We also need to record the decisions that the person makes in a decision-making agreement. In Chapter 3 we heard some of Louisa's story; here is her decision-making agreement (Figure 4.6).

Decision Making Profile				
How Meg likes her information	How to present choice to Meg	How can you help Meg understand	When are the best times to ask Meg to make a decision	When is it not a good time to ask Meg to make decisions
Visual – must be the real thing not photos or pictures.	Use Meg's name at the end of each point. Gain her attention – eye contact. Pause – allow time between options. Avoid open questions – look for 'yes' or 'no' answers from Meg. No more than two options at a time.	Speak clearly and slowly – short sentences. Repeat Meg's words back to her. One piece of information at a time. Avoid questions. Summarise what you have understood back to Meg.	When Meg is talkative.	Not early morning – i.e. before breakfast and not after teatime.

Figure 4.5 Meg's decision-making profile

Decision Making Agreement

Decision	How Louisa must be involved and who can help	Who makes the final decision?
Using a straw and lid on beaker to drink (when Louisa can't swallow properly) or not, whether she uses the blender to purée her food.	Dietician and GP talk it through with Louisa not support staff.	Louisa does, after taking into account advice I have been given.
Where to sleep – bed or recliner chair.	Physiotherapist explains any problems that may arise as a result of sleeping regularly on the recliner.	Louisa.
To go out on her own to the shops.	Louisa talks it through with her son and daughter.	Louisa.

Figure 4.6 Louisa's decision-making agreement

Once we know how much choice and control someone has in her life now, as described in their decision-making agreement, the next question must be 'What can we do to increase it?'

This can mean looking at the decision-making agreement and asking:

- What would it take for the person to have more control in the important decisions in her life?

- What other decisions would the person like to have more control over?

These are the actions and decisions for answering those questions with Louisa:

1. Joanne and Michael will talk through situations with Louisa as they arise as this really supports Louisa to feel more confident in decision making.

2. Gill and Louisa are using *Living Well* (Sanderson and Lancashire County Council 2010) at Louisa's request to help her think about living well in the now, and to think and plan around her end-of-life wishes.

3. Louisa and her Admiral nurse are going to develop a sheet exploring 'how best to support Louisa to be involved in all decision making and who else to involve in which decisions'. The relationship circle will inform their thinking on who in Louisa's life are the best people to be involved in specific decisions. This will be used to advise everyone supporting Louisa in her involvement in decision making.

Enabling people to have more choice and control requires us to understand why they have so little of it to begin with. Here are some possible reasons (there are lots more):

- Staff are not giving people opportunities to make decisions themselves.

- People are not in control of their own services.

- People have few choices because they don't know what else could be possible.

- Staff don't understand the ways that people try to communicate and see their behaviour as 'challenging', not as communication.

- Staff don't have or take the time to listen.

- Staff don't expect people to make choices.

- Staff see their role as taking care of people and looking after them, not enabling people to make choices. There is an ingrained task-focused culture.

- Staff don't know how to enable people to make choices.

- It is easier to do things quickly for people than to take the time to support them to make choices.

Once we know the possible reasons, we can then look at potential solutions. Personal budgets directly address the first two reasons; training and support to use person-centred thinking tools such as the communication charts and decision-making agreements are very helpful; and you will also see the importance of staff understanding their role as supporting people to have as much choice and control as possible. Personalisation requires a cultural change from a task-orientated ethos to one that values what matters most to the people being supported and focuses on relationships and citizenship.

Decision Making Agreement

Decisions in Jane's life	How Jane must be involved and who else can help	Who makes the final decision?
What Jane eats.	Offered a choice of two low-sugar meals and desserts.	Jane.
If Jane sticks to her special diet – low-sugar due to diabetes (see care plan for detail).	District nurse tells her daily what her blood sugar levels are.	Jane.
What time Jane has her meals.	Not negotiable in this setting unless Jane wants a sandwich.	The home managers.
When Jane goes out and where she goes to.	That Jane is listened to when she says she would like to go out. Discuss with her if it is not possible – explaining and setting a day and time when it will be possible. Enter this on the calendar on Jane's bedroom wall.	The home managers.
Recruitment of new staff.	Jane is included on the interview panel to give her view.	The interview panel on a majority decision.
What time to get up.	Ask Jane before she goes to bed what time she would like to get up in the morning.	Jane.
Bath or shower?	Ask Jane which she would prefer.	Jane.
What to wear.	Show Jane a range of clothes from her wardrobe.	Jane decides what colours and which clothes.
How much money to spend from her allowance and what on.	Paula, Jane's daughter, controls her allowance and will discuss with Jane what she needs.	Paula with input from Jane.

Figure 4.7 Jane's decision-making agreement

Here is another example. Jane lives in a residential service supporting older people. She has recently been diagnosed with Alzheimer's disease and the staff team used decision-making agreements to develop a picture of how empowered Jane is and to explore how they can enhance and maintain the choice and control she has in her life as the condition progresses (Figure 4.7).

Decision making for the future – end-of-life wishes

Person-centred thinking can also be used in decision making for end-of-life wishes and advance directives, which set out how a person wants to be cared for as they come to the end of their life, or if they lose mental capacity.

Here, Sally talks about how she approached this with her mum, Audree, and the role that person-centred thinking tools played. *Living Well: Thinking and Planning for the End of Your Life* is a booklet of person-centred thinking tools to help people plan for the end of their life (Sanderson and Lancashire County Council 2010).

Audree's end-of-life wishes

I would like to tell you about my mum, Audree. Without doubt the biggest influence in my life, she has always taken an interest in her children's lives and to this day she still professes how proud she is of us and is there to support and advise us in whatever we are involved in. From her I have also learned that sometimes you have to put others' needs ahead of your own, and she has done this every day of her life for her family, friends and anyone who needs a helping hand.

My mother's strength seemed to be unbreakable during hard times. This was particularly evident when my father suddenly died and she was left with two very distressed teenage girls and an extremely demanding job with no home or security. Her determination to care and love for her family pushed her to regaining everything that we lost. She worked tirelessly as a head teacher in a large primary school where her skill and inspiration as a teacher had a huge impact on the children she taught. Several of her students still remain in contact with her even though she has been retired for 15 years and moved 300 miles from the schools she taught in. However, my mother never let her work get in the way of our relationship and always had time to comfort a broken heart, celebrate our successes or just sit and talk for no particular reason. I always admired her open mind, compassion and great sense of humour.

At 79, Mum fell and broke her leg. Unfortunately, this break went undiagnosed for a year and by the time it was diagnosed the damage to her leg was irreversible and she had lost the ability to walk. The decision was taken by professionals to place her in a care home. It was a terrible experience for Mum and she lost the will to live; she became a shadow of her former self as she was being eaten away with bed sores and depression. Then one day I went into the home to visit Mum and she was lying flat in bed choking on her own vomit. Her call button had been hidden in a drawer and I am sure that without my intervention she would have died. I could stand it no longer and fought for her to come home with a personal budget. Within two months her inner self was healing nicely, the sores were gone and I no longer had the guilt of leaving her in a care home that was failing her in every way.

My mother is now 82. She struggles with mobility – in fact, she can only use her arms (which is just as well as she can maintain her treats – smoking and a daily glass of wine!) – and dementia is now taking over her sharp mind. However, her spirit still shines through and she is dealing with it with the elegance, humour and courage she has displayed all of her life.

I now have power of attorney for her so I am able to make decisions for her and with her. This is a serious responsibility and it is vital that I make accurate choices. I admit I made assumptions based on the fact that I know her so well. I attended a workshop with Helen (Sanderson) and she talked about *Living Well*, a guide to help you think about and record what is important to you now and what you want in the future (planning for the end of your life). I didn't think it would help me learn more about my mum, but I thought it would help me to capture exactly what she needed and wanted to happen now and in the future, and then I could share it with the rest of our family.

I was a little frightened about approaching some of the questions regarding the end of life and funeral planning, but I suppressed my fear and carried on regardless. I made us a coffee and we just started talking about her life, capturing her important memories in the booklet. We really enjoyed it and I was surprised at some of the funny stories and magical moments that Mum shared with me that I had never heard before. The next time I visited, Mum immediately said, 'Can we do more of that book?' so we looked at the relationship circle and this sparked new and different stories about people Mum had known and loved. Talking about friends made Mum want to talk to some that she hadn't spoken to for a while and she asked me to phone my godmother and write to her old next-door neighbour.

Each time I visited Mum we did a little more. I found the section about 'what is important to me now and how best to support me' invaluable. Mum has very clear ideas about how she wants to live her life and it made it so much easier for her various personal assistants to read a concise account of what Mum truly wanted and how they could support her best. It was very reassuring when we got to the 'working and not working' section, as there was very little on the 'not working' side and it was apparent that Mum was happy with her life.

When we discussed the serious subject of 'hopes and fears', Mum was very clear that her absolute fear was to be forced back into a care home. This information proved invaluable. Recently, Mum had a continuing health care assessment and I was told that without doubt she would be happier and healthier in a care home. I was adamant that Mum would hate it, but they were firm that she couldn't possibly know what was good for her. So I showed the panel the booklet that proved exactly what she feared the most and consequently she has remained at home but with additional night cover.

We carried on with the booklet little by little, chatting and laughing but recording really important information. When we started 'planning for the end of your life', it was me that found it difficult. The thought of Mum not being here is heart-wrenching and emotional, but because of the way the booklet progresses Mum was fine. The booklet eases you naturally into thinking about what next and she was keen to carry on and I am so, so glad we did. This section threw up the most astounding information. I said earlier that I know my mother so well, but that led me to make inaccurate assumptions, and if we hadn't discussed end-of-life planning I would have got it so wrong. Through our discussions I discovered that not only would I have missed inviting key people to the funeral, I would have buried her in the wrong place, with the wrong people!! That is a pretty serious mistake to make.

When we had finished the booklet we realised how important it will become because Mum's dementia will only get worse. This booklet will contain her living wishes so that when she can no longer express her needs, they will be recorded clearly as a reminder of what she really wants to happen to her. I don't want to think about her death, but at least I now know I will get things as right as possible and she will live out her life the way she wants it. When she is gone we will also have a wonderful booklet of memories for us to share with children, grandchildren and, who knows, great-grandchildren. I have now shared Mum's wishes with the rest of the family and they are also relieved as they too would have got it all wrong.

The process of completing this booklet with Mum also gave us time together. It made me sit down and spend time with her, talking and laughing, which sometimes got forgotten within my hectic life, so for that I am so grateful. (See Figures 4.8 and 4.9.)

What do I want to add as I think about the end of my life?

What I want	What I don't want	My family's view
Where I want to die		
I want to be at home.	I don't want to die in a hospital or a care home.	We will support Mum to stay at home.
About my funeral (music, readings, flowers, etc.)		
Frank Sinatra – Young at Heart, Paris Angelicus, Sally to do a reading, freesias.	Nothing religious.	We will make sure Mum gets what she wants.
About being buried or cremated (clothes, hair, makeup, jewellery)		
I really don't mind.	Nothing valuable.	
About the scattering of my ashes		
I want to be buried with Les and Mum and Dad.	Is to be on my own.	We will ensure Mum gets her wishes.
About what people do after my funeral (e.g. a celebration, memorial)		
Celebration at home with lots of food and wine.	To do nothing.	We will organise it.
About a gravestone or marker for my ashes or burial place		
To be added to Les' headstone with words about being a wife, mother and grandmother.	Lots of flowers. I want donations for a paralympics.	We agree with Mum and will organise it.
What else is important to me		
I want Sally and boys to be with me at the end.	To be alone.	

Figure 4.8 Completed page from Audree's Living Well:
Thinking and Planning for the End of Your Life

How would I like to be remembered?

> I would like to have a Trust Fund set up called
> The Audree Shephard Trust which will sponsor a
> paralympian to attend and take part in the Olympics.
>
> I want notification of my death to be in the
> Westmorland Gazette and the Biggleswade Chronicle.
>
> On the anniversary of my death I want you to open
> a bottle of Champagne, look at family photos and
> remember the good times we had as a family.
>
> Keep my autobiography safe for my great-
> grandchildren to read and learn about me.

*Figure 4.9 Completed page from Audree's Living Well:
Thinking and Planning for the End of Your Life*

Tough decisions?

Sally's account of working with her mother to identify her end-of-life wishes shows that even the most painful subjects can be discussed and decisions made. Many people feel a great sense of relief when major decisions have been written down, knowing that their wishes will be respected. Of course, many people with dementia are less able to articulate their choices and decisions than Audree was at this point, and the people closest to them will need to be involved in discussions, perhaps over a long period of time, and final decisions.

In the next chapter we discuss another major area of people's lives – *who* supports them.

Chapter 5

Matching Staff and Clarifying Responsibilities

The ability to create and develop relationships with others is crucial to our well-being... There is nothing about dementia that changes this: indeed, the increasing dependency on others which inevitably accompanies dementia emphasises, rather than detracts from, the need for supportive relationships with others.

Nuffield Council on Bioethics (2009)

The biggest influence on the quality of life of people living with dementia is their relationship with the people who support them. When this is working well, the carer knows what matters to the person, understands how they communicate and make decisions, and supports them in exactly the way they want to be supported, balancing what is important *to* them with what is important *for* them. To improve the quality of people's lives, we can go even further than that. Many people think that enhancing the quality of life for people with dementia is about amazing buildings and excellent hotel services. These may be important to some people, but the quality of relationships is more important to most. However clear the information is about what matters to the person and her opportunities to make decisions, if she is not supported by people she likes, and who like her, life will be miserable. Staff and volunteers in homecare and residential care are typically organised and deployed in a way that does not take into account relationships or shared interests. This means that staff don't always have the opportunity of working with someone they like, and the likelihood of ending up with people who like each other, with interests in common, is then random at best.

A good match is a win–win. When we take into account a staff member's characteristics and interests, as well as their skills and experience, we are more likely to get a match that is enjoyable for everyone. When staff enjoy their work, they are more likely to stay longer in the role; this increases the stability for the individual and decreases staff turnover for the organisation. It could be argued that we are less likely to see issues of abuse and neglect when we pay good attention to matching people well. This approach is also more likely to help to deliver personalised services rather than 'covering shifts': 'The quality of the match is one of the most powerful determinants of quality of life for people who are dependent on others for support and the single greatest determinant of turnover among those paid to provide services' (Smull and Sanderson 2005, p.21).

This chapter looks at ways of getting a good match between people living with dementia and the staff and volunteers who support them, and, when we have got a good match, how to make sure that staff responsibilities are clear.

Getting a good match – the matching tool

The matching tool has four columns. The first is the support that the person wants and needs, then the skills required to support them, followed by personality characteristics and then shared common interests. The most important part of this is the section where personality characteristics are recorded.

Hilda lives in the North-West and has early-onset dementia. Her family are looking for support for her to stay at home. The characteristics of the staff who would be the best match for Hilda are shown in Figure 5.1.

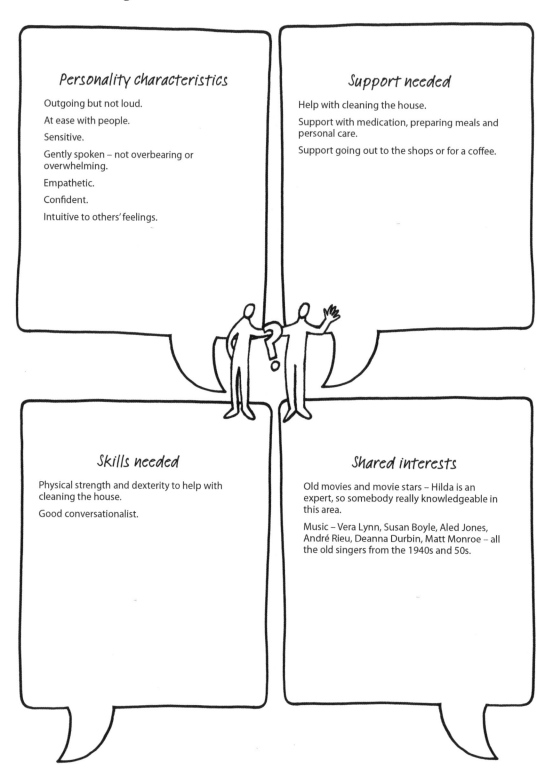

Figure 5.1 Matching support to Hilda

Using this person-centred thinking tool should ensure that you list the skills that someone providing support needs in order to meet what is both important *to* and important *for* the person in need of support. This is a minimum expectation. Matching characteristics is also crucial. If the person cannot directly tell you the characteristics of the people with whom she gets on best, here are some questions that are useful:

- Who is the person closest to? What characteristics do they have in common?

- With whom does the person have the most 'good days'?

- Is there anyone whose presence helps create 'bad days'?

- What does this tell you about the characteristics of the support person?

This person-centred thinking tool can be used to match existing staff within a team to particular individuals, to recruit new people to a team, or to recruit personal assistants or find volunteers. It is easier to develop good matches when the staff or volunteers also have one-page profiles. In Winifred's story, Lisa, the manager, paid attention to shared interests as well as skills in matching her with Beryl.

Winifred's story

Winifred is a wonderful, loving personality who brightens the room when she enters it. She lives in a residential service with 43 other people who are living with dementia. Winifred's daughters and the team recognised that Winifred was feeling lost at times and so Lisa and Gill spent an hour with Winifred and her two daughters, Maureen and Bernie, to develop her one-page profile. Her daughters described her as a 'real home-maker' and a good day was tidying and cleaning the house. This was clearly very important to Winifred. They decided together that what would make her happiest was to be involved in cleaning and tidying, in her home at Bruce Lodge. The next decision was who she wanted to support her.

As well as supporting everyone who lived at Bruce Lodge to do a one-page profile, Gill and Lisa supported all the staff to do their own one-page profiles as well. This included Beryl, the housekeeper, and Lisa thought that Beryl would be the natural choice to support Winifred to get involved in the tidying and cleaning. Lisa turned out to be right. Now you can hear Winifred singing aloud as she polishes, mops, washes up and carries out the chores she did so routinely in her own home before she moved here. The increase in well-being is clear to see. Maureen and Bernie have noticed the change this has made to their mother, in that she is happier, chatting more, using fuller sentences, is sleeping better and is generally 'more alive'.

Once we know the best person or people to provide support, the next task is to clarify their roles and responsibilities.

Clarifying roles and responsibilities

A powerful way to help staff to be clear about their roles and responsibilities in supporting people is through Charles Handy's *doughnut* (Handy 1994). He uses a doughnut to help people to think about what is core to their role or task, and where they can be creative and flexible (Figure 5.2).

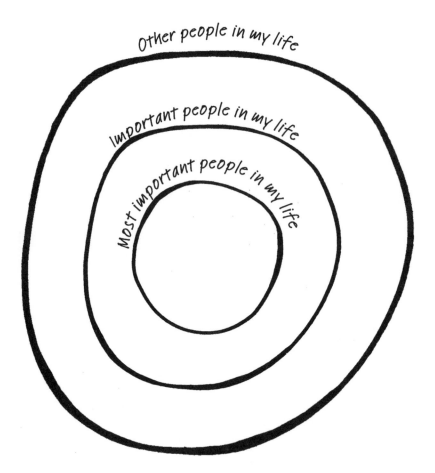

Figure 5.2 The doughnut

The heart of the doughnut – the core – contains everything that must be done in that job or role if you are to succeed. In a formal job description, these are listed as your duties. The next ring is our opportunity to go beyond the bounds of duty, to experiment and learn. Michael Smull developed the doughnut to include a third circle, to identify areas that are not the responsibilities of staff:

- The first ring is the inner core, which consists of the core responsibilities of staff or people providing support.

- The next ring covers areas where staff need to exercise their own judgement and be creative. These are areas where people must make decisions, problem-solve and creatively think about possibilities and potential.

- The final ring indicates areas beyond the scope of the staff member's role and responsibilities. All roles have limits and boundaries, some of which are formally in place and some of which are informal – for example, family preferences or respect for cultural differences.

You need to know what is important to and for someone before you begin to use the doughnut tool to clarify the roles of staff in specific situations. Using the doughnut ring is a great way to explain responsibilities to people but hard to use in practice, so we use the same headings in columns (see Figure 5.3).

Ken is a former professional footballer with Stockport County, a fun-loving man with dementia who, for the last three years, has lived in a care home. Ken's family sat down with him and some of the team members who knew him best to discuss what they could do to help Ken, who appeared to have lost his sense of fun and zest for life. They had several conversations together and developed a one-page profile with Ken. What emerged as really important to Ken were things such as 'sharing his Stockport County memorabilia and old photos', 'watching football on TV' and 'having people around him to enjoy banter with'. Ken will always seek people out and be 'amongst it', as he says. Based on this learning, they began to think about what it would take to support Ken to watch Stockport play a home game and it was soon arranged. After going to a couple of games, a number of things emerged that had to happen to make it a good experience for Ken. The team developed a doughnut to capture these things in terms of the staff team's core responsibilities, where they could use judgement and creativity to extend the experience even further for Ken, and what was not their responsibility (Figure 5.3). Charles Handy (1994) also talks about two types of errors that staff can make: Type 1 and Type 2.

Type 1 errors simply mean getting it wrong – an error in the core responsibilities of the doughnut, where someone did not do what they should. Once, for example, Ken's staff had not stayed until the final whistle because they wanted to get away from the ground before it became really crowded as all the fans left. Ken was incredibly upset. He didn't make a fuss about it but mentioned every day for the week after the game that 'it is just not right to leave a game before the final whistle'. It was apparent this had really spoiled the experience for him. Now we know that this is a core responsibility for staff supporting Ken to see a game.

Type 2 errors occur when the full possibilities of a situation have not been explored. An example might include not considering what else could be done to achieve a better outcome than would be expected by just delivering the core responsibilities. In Ken's doughnut, an example would be having a drink in a local pub. When the staff member supporting Ken did this, she was amazed that in this home fans' pub a number of the fans recognised Ken as an ex-player and saw him as a hero. Everybody wanted to buy Ken a drink and he visibly grew as he basked in this wonderful atmosphere. Had the staff member not used her judgement based on her football knowledge, these connections would never have been made. Such a missed opportunity is what Handy calls a Type 2 error.

Using the doughnut also helps to create a culture of learning and accountability, rather than fear and blame, by enabling people to think clearly about responsibilities and possibilities, and delineating who is responsible for what. This enables staff to be creative without anxiety, knowing what would be understood as Type 1 errors, but also aware that not exploring possibilities creatively is a Type 2 error. It is well known that one of the big stressors in work is lack of clarity as to what people expect from staff. Therefore it is possible and likely that creating this clarity through using the doughnut could have an impact on reducing staff stress and increasing retention.

Clear boundaries are also very important when people have different roles in a person's life. Hilda's family employs a homecare organisation to support her. They developed a doughnut that reflected what the family saw as their role, and what is core to that, and what was core for the homecare service and where they could be flexible and creative. This 'split doughnut' looks at how to support Hilda well, and the different roles and responsibilities that the family and the homecare provider have (Figure 5.4).

In the next chapter we turn our attention to another key staffing issue: how we can move from person-centred information and knowing what matters to someone to change what is not working in their life.

Responsibilities

Core responsibilities

- Book transport to get to and from the match.
- Get to the stadium for 2.15pm.
- Buy a programme.
- Have a hot chocolate while standing at the snack bar.
- Be in match seat for 2.45pm.
- Stay until the final whistle.
- Support Ken in connecting with others.

Use judgement and creativity

- Try using public transport.
- Having a drink in a local pub after the match.
- How you celebrate with Ken if they win.
- How you support him around bad results.
- Going through the programme at half-time.
- Chatting with other fans, seeking natural networks.
- Finding opportunities for Ken to be involved in community projects with the club.

Not our responsibility

- Whether his team wins or loses.

Figure 5.3 Ken's doughnut to support him to watch football matches

	Core responsibilities	Where we can be creative and use our own judgment	Not our responsibility
Hilda, Gill and family	To talk to the manager if there is anything that we are unhappy with, or want to compliment the staff on.	Whether we phone or email the manager. Whether we say anything directly to the person themselves.	How the manager addresses issues with staff.
Home care provider	To match two staff to Hilda based on what she needs, and her preferences.	How you find the best match.	To ask the family to update the one-page profile.
Homecare provider	To ensure that staff turn up on time on the right day. Never to provide other staff than the two Hilda knows. Ensure that staff support Hilda in the way described on her one-page profile.	How you ensure that staff are delivering the service required. What you ask staff to record about their visits. How staff record their learning. How the one-page profile is kept updated to reflect learning.	Organising the cleaners; Merrymaids. To check Hilda's medication.
Support Worker	Read and follow the information captured on Hilda's one page profile. To go to Sainsburys and support Hilda as described on her one-page profile.	How you spend your time with Hilda through conversation with her, she may not want to pay her papers or go to the village for bread some weeks. If you have a cup of tea and biscuit/ cake with Hilda in her home. How you put Hilda at ease and develop a good relationship.	

Figure 5.4 Roles and responsibilities in supporting Hilda (split doughnut)

Chapter 6

Acting on What Is Working and Not Working

> A person-centred review is a person-centred approach to the annual reviews required in all services.
>
> *Department of Health (2010a)*

> A person-centred review can create significant change in how people live their lives, based on what people want to achieve – it makes a difference.
>
> *Wendy, member of the Transforming Adult Social Care*
> *Reference Group (Department of Health 2010a)*

In the book so far we have looked at different ways of gathering information for a one-page profile, how people make decisions and how to get the best match between the person and staff, to ensure that people living with dementia have personalised support and as much choice and control in their lives as possible. But we must not stop there. Central to personalisation is moving from 'knowing' to acting on information about what is important to and for a person, and how much control he has in his life. If we do not do this, we simply create what Michael Smull describes as 'good paperwork', instead of working with people to enable them to have 'good lives' (Sanderson and Lewis 2012).

Working and not working from different perspectives

As soon as there is enough information about someone recorded in a one-page profile, we need to use the person-centred thinking tool *working and not working* to build an action plan to make sure that the support that people are getting works for them. In this way, *working and not working* serves as a bridge between what was learned about what matters to the person and how to support them well and action planning (Sanderson and Lewis 2012).

In Chapter 3, we heard about Edie and saw her communication charts. The manager arranged a meeting with Edie, her son and daughter, and two staff members who knew Edie really well. They spent an hour together over a cup of tea discussing Edie's one-page profile, which they had developed several months before, and began to think about what was working and not working and captured this on to the *working/not working* analysis. They then developed actions to change the things that were not working.

Here is Edie's one-page profile (Figure 6.1), and then what is working and not working from her family's perspective, our best guess at Edie's perspective and the staff's perspective as well (Figure 6.2).

Edie's one-page profile

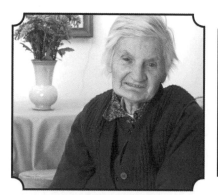

What people appreciate about Edie

- Her beautiful voice.
- Cuts to the chase – says it how it is.
- Great laugh.
- Very honest talker.

What is important to Edie

- Barbara, her daughter, Bernard, her son, and Christopher who visit often.
- Hearing about what's going on and who is doing what from her family and around the home.
- Her handbag – it must never leave her side. Edie sleeps with her handbag by her pillow – it must never be moved from her.
- Always knowing where her money is and that Christopher is looking after everything.
- People-watching – Edie will often spend time content in simply watching others.
- Sitting outdoors in the garden when it is sunny, but Edie is a home bird and not keen on going out beyond the garden.
- Watching animal programmes on TV.
- Having her hair done and looking nice and smart.
- To be acknowledged and complimented often on how lovely she looks.
- Having her nails manicured and varnished.
- Bananas and chocolates are always welcomed – she loves milk chocolate.
- To reminisce and share her stories is a must.
- To sing; Edie has a beautiful voice – she is always singing. She loves music – especially Viennese piano.
- To have her tea (rather than coffee) served in a china cup (medium brew, two sugars and milk) with biscuits.
- To always choose her clothes – she takes great pride in her appearance.
- Not sitting alone in her bedroom – being out and about in the home.
- Daisy the cat.

How best to support Edie

- Edie avoids going to bed as she doesn't recognise that this is home. Reassure her it is fine to sleep here as it is dark outside. Then feels easier about going to bed.
- Edie worries that the home is under surveillance and the police are coming – we are trying to work out how to support Edie well around this.
- Edie is not comfortable in large groups. She has always avoided getting involved with groups of women.
- Compliment Edie on her appearance often.
- Never move Edie's handbag away from her.
- Give Edie reassurance if she is upset and agitated looking for her mum (Minnie) and her dad. Reminisce with her about them.
- Edie will believe she is in her mother's house and wants to know who all these other people are. Sitting and asking her to tell her stories from her childhood days eases her anxiety.
- Edie will worry about having her hair done. Because she doesn't know who is paying, reassure her that Christopher has paid for it.
- Explore opportunities and activities with Edie that will increase her well-being and occupy her mind to decrease her anxieties.
- Reassure Edie that Christopher looks after her money and ensures everything is paid.
- Edie will call out 'kidnap' if she is out in town and has had enough. Reassure her you will go back home immediately.
- Be aware that Edie takes her walking frame into bed and gets comfy under the duvet, as she is fearful somebody will steal it. Leave Edie be; she is quite safe and comfortable with the walking frame in the bed.

Figure 6.1 Edie's one-page profile

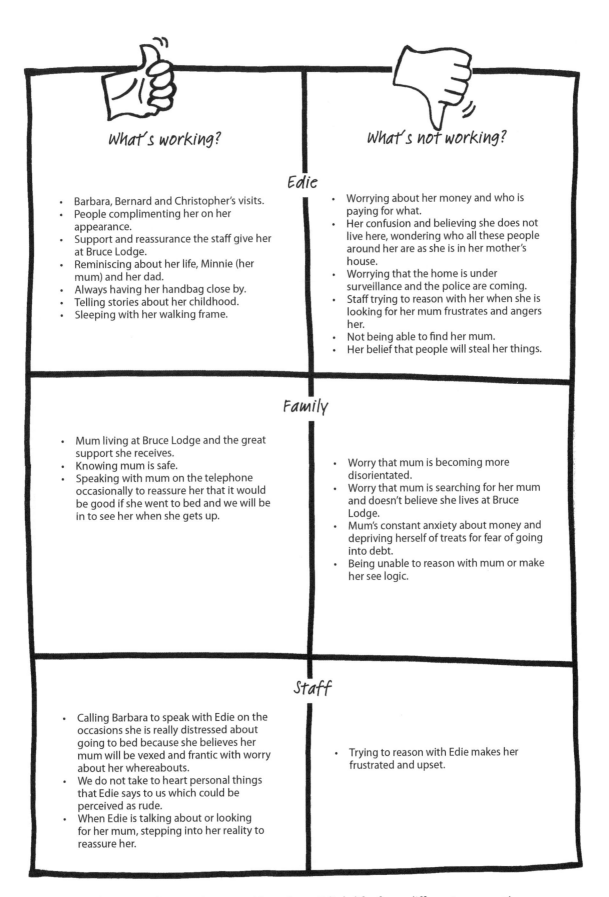

Figure 6.2 What is working and not working about Edie's life, from different perspectives

Figure 6.3 shows the actions that came from looking at what is working and not working for Edie, from different perspectives.

Who	Will do what	By when
Joan	Arrange for a session on the team meeting agenda to support team members to develop communication charts, to help us support Edie more consistently.	August 5th
Sue and Liz	Spot the opportunities and coach staff on a day-to-day basis in making best guesses about what Edie is telling us and develop communication charts or add learning to the one-page profile.	From August 5th
Sue	Will ask the training section to come in and help staff recognise that we need to seek out the feelings which lie behind Edie's behaviours. For example, when Edie says she needs to go to her mum, she may well be feeling insecure and unloved. We need to shift the team's thinking by asking what good support would look like around this.	August 18th
Joan	Invite Edie's family to the session outlined above.	August 5th
Barbara (Edie's daughter)	Will ask Christopher to make a list of how much money Edie has spent each week and how much she has left to spend and go through it with Edie every Sunday, reassuring her she has enough left for the things she wants, such as getting her hair done.	August 5th

Figure 6.3 Actions from what is working and not working for Edie

The *working/not working* person-centred thinking tool is powerful in three ways:

1. It is a simple way to analyse what is happening in someone's life, whether what is important to her is present in her life, and whether she is being supported in the way that makes sense to her. Problems surface where there are areas of disagreement in people's lives. By looking at what is working and not working from different perspectives, it is clear where there is agreement and where there is difference. The different perspectives would usually be the person themselves, family and staff. Where the person is supported by professionals – for example, a social worker or physiotherapist – their perspective would also be included. Looking at a situation from different perspectives enables people to see things 'all the way round' and to stand in different people's shoes. *Working and not working* from different perspectives contains two of the core principles of negotiation. When you get each person's perspective on paper, they feel listened to. When you tease situations apart in enough detail, you can find areas of agreement and this enables you to start on 'common ground' (Smull and Sanderson 2005).

2. It looks at areas of disagreement in the context of what people agree is going well. This is an important starting point for discussion and change. It also gives providers an opportunity to acknowledge and appreciate what is going well, which can so often be overlooked.

3. It prevents us from inadvertently changing aspects of a person's life that are working for them.

You can look together with the person and their family at what is working and not working at any time. One way to do this more formally, on an annual basis, is through a person-centred review.

Reflecting on how things are going and making change – person-centred reviews

A person-centred review is a meeting that combines two person-centred thinking skills and tools: an understanding of the balance between *important to* and *important for* the person with what is *working and not working* from different perspectives. The purpose is to create shared actions for change, based on reflection on and analysis of what is working and not working for the person and others. Person-centred reviews also provide enough information to start a one-page profile or update a profile that is already being used.

A person-centred review brings together people who are providing support from different roles or places, with family and friends. It places the person who is being supported firmly at the centre, even if they no longer use words to communicate.

Mary's person-centred review

Mary, now in her 80s, took up a career as a nurse, training as a midwife and a theatre sister. She emigrated to Canada following a couple of years in New York where she met and married Bert Bailey in 1956. They had two daughters, Nancy and Jennifer (Jenny). She returned to England with her children following the break-up of her marriage and brought the girls up alone, remaining single for the rest of her life. She retired from nursing at 68 and went on to volunteer as a carer and support the work of the local church in Waterloo, Liverpool. Mary spent a lot of time with her daughters and five grandchildren. Nancy moved to Australia and Jennifer remained in England with her two children, Adam and Katie. Mary remains in constant contact with her family. She was diagnosed with Alzheimer's in her mid-70s.

Mary has always been a stickler for good manners and etiquette, and has a strong work ethic. Her Christian faith and church have always played a part in her life, providing spiritual comfort and a community in later life. Mary has always found herself in a primary care role through her work, home life and voluntary work with older people, providing aromatherapy and reflexology services. She has never really enjoyed large groups; although confident on the outside, Mary was always a shy person, enjoying the company of one or two people. When in large groups, such as a party, Mary was always more comfortable as the hostess or helping in the kitchen rather than mingling with the crowd.

Mary has lived for the last three years in an extra care housing scheme and she also attends their day service. Her condition deteriorated significantly after a fall when she broke her kneecap in June 2012, which resulted in a three-month stay in hospital. After a hard-fought battle with Continuing Health Care funders, discharge planners, clinical and social work staff who all deemed Mary was best placed in a nursing home, Mary returned to her own home in October 2012. This was made possible by the belief of the family and the support team that the best possible outcome for Mary was to return to her home, to be supported by people who knew her and who would ensure those things that mattered to her were present in her life, and that she was supported in a way that worked for her.

Following the delivery of specialist equipment to meet Mary's needs, the discharge papers were signed. At this time Mary was assessed as requiring two staff to transfer her and the use of a hoist at all times. She was not able to use a knife and fork or take fluid independently, so she was deemed as requiring constant support at meal times; she was also doubly incontinent.

Mary had a person-centred review with the family and her staff team at home, using the headings shown in Figure 6.4 to explore how her support was going.

The social worker called a review after Mary had been at home for six weeks. They used the person-centred review process. Jenny decided who to invite on Mary's behalf. She invited two of the extra care staff (who support her in her flat) and two of the day service staff, as well as the social worker and Gill who facilitated the review. The person-centred review took place in Mary's flat. The process naturally begins with introductions, so Gill asked everyone to introduce themselves, in relation to their role in Mary's life.

At this stage, a typical review would involve social workers and professionals reading their reports. However, in a person-centred review the person shares their own perspective and then everyone else, including family and friends, adds their views and information is shared and built together. In Mary's review, Gill wrote information on flipcharts. Another way to do this is round a table, using A4 sheets of paper with a question written on the top of each sheet. These are circulated round the table for people to add their information. The way that information is shared is decided with the person, taking into account the number of people coming to the review and where it will be held. The aim is to create a comfortable atmosphere that gives everyone an equal opportunity to have their say, and for this information to be recorded.

Information is recorded about the following questions:

- What do we appreciate about the person?

- What is important to the person now?

- What is important to the person for the future?

- What does the person need to stay healthy and safe, and to be supported well?

- What questions do we need to answer?

- What is working and not working from different perspectives?

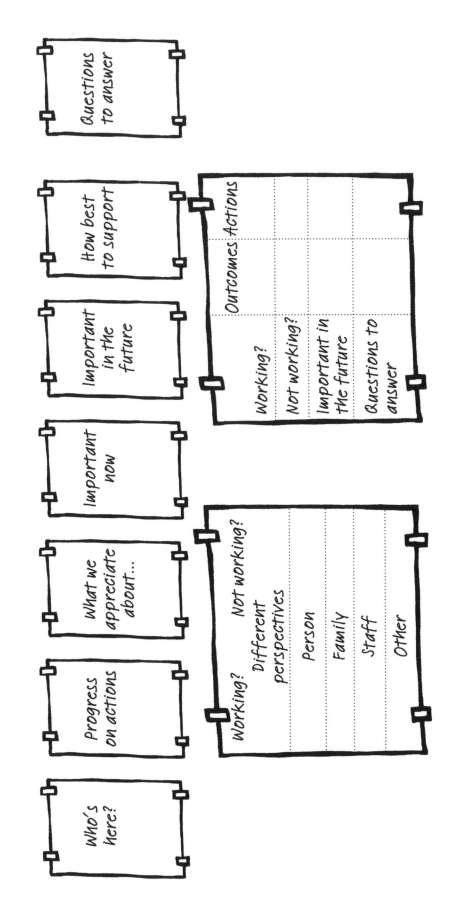

Figure 6.4 The headings in a person-centred review

The 'what questions do we need to answer?' is where people ensure that statutory requirements are addressed. It is also a place to record any questions or issues that the person or their supporters want to work on or work out. In Mary's case, the social worker had some key questions that she wanted answers to.

Once the information has been shared and recorded, the next stage is to use it to explore any differences in opinion and to generate actions. Actions are agreed that keep what is working for the person and change what is not working for them. In this way, the person-centred review makes it more likely that the person will have what is important to them in their life and move towards the future they want. You may be able to address what is not working for people within the current service and resources. You may need to use other person-centred thinking skills to find out what needs to be done differently (see pages 85–87).

The process also uses this person-centred information to build a detailed person-centred description. This differs from a one-page profile simply by being more detailed.

In Mary's review, Gill asked the following questions to help to get to actions:

- What needs to happen to make sure that what is working in Mary's life keeps happening?

- What needs to happen to change what is not working for Mary?

- How can we address each of the 'questions to answer'? What else do we need to learn?

- What can we do together to enable Mary to move towards what is important in the future?

Here is the information that everyone contributed at Mary's review:

What others appreciate about Mary

- Her beautiful manners.

- A lovely smile.

- A real lady.

- Dry sense of humour and doesn't suffer fools.

- Mary doesn't need to say anything – one of her looks says it all.

Important to Mary

- To maintain her spiritual belief through Christian rituals and celebrations. Singing hymns, watching services on TV and taking part in services.

- Spending time with her family. Mary has regular contact with her daughter, Jennifer, and grandchildren, Adam and Katie.

- Conversations about her experiences when she was nursing and when she was a midwife.

- Listening to music – 1940s and 1950s. She loves the Glen Miller Orchestra, Gilbert and Sullivan opera, popular theatre music and religious music.

- That others have a laugh and a joke with her – silly dancing, facial expressions and generally 'acting the fool'.

- Going through magazines about gardening, animals or household things, talking about daily activities such as shopping and cooking.

- Mary enjoys the closeness of people she feels safe with, holding hands, hugs, smiles and general chat.

- Sitting where she can see all the comings and goings; Mary loves to people-watch.

- People acknowledging Mary by greeting her with a smile, addressing her by name and making eye contact with a big smile.

- Mary loves to help and feel she is involved. She loves nothing more than assisting others.

- Mary enjoys massage to her hands/arms, having trained in reflexology following retirement. Asking her to do this for others will give her back the feeling of doing for others, which was extremely important to her throughout her life.

- To sort and fold laundry or arrange items – for example, putting away cutlery.

- Being complimented! Chat about her clothes. She must look smart and takes pride in her appearance. It is important to her that clothes are neat and tidy; marks, loose threads and missing buttons can cause distraction.

- Mary hates to be cold, so must always wear a cardigan and something warm on her feet; when sitting, she has to have a warm cover over her legs.

- To have items close to her that provide comfort – for example, her blanket and handbag. Having her cuddly animals such as her cats close by is a must.

- Mary adores seeing children play; she will come alive when babies and small children are around.

- Animals have always been a large part of Mary's life as she grew up with pet dogs and cats, and she enjoys watching the birds or petting domestic animals. Mary will also watch wildlife programmes and programmes where animals feature.

What is important to Mary in the future

- To continue to live in her own place with people she knows.

How to support Mary

- Ensure her family are kept updated on what Mary has been doing to support good conversations.

- Mary is uncomfortable with males in close proximity and should not have males for personal care, although she is happy for support from her grandson and is extremely close to him.

- Make sure that you are in Mary's sightline before you speak and go up close so that she can hear you; use simple signs with speech to give her visual clues. Use her name if you are directing conversation to her.

- Provide opportunities for Mary to 'help' and feel purpose. This can be achieved through simple activities – for example, asking 'Can you fold that for me?' or 'Could you wash those dishes?' Using exaggerated praise really boosts her self-worth.

- Mary enjoys the company of others but not large groups as she cannot follow the conversation and will withdraw.

- Mary is very tuned into tone of voice, facial expression and approach, so it is important that support is provided in a calm, patient manner as she hates being rushed.

- Mary is polite and manners have always been important to her. She does not like loud offensive language. Be mindful of this when supporting Mary to sit with other people in the day service.

- Mary gets cold quickly and must be kept warm.

- Mary relates well to people who are outwardly loving and friendly towards her; she reads faces so will pick up easily on tension.

- Show Mary lots of love and attention, smile and engage in conversation. Never just walk past her without acknowledgement.

- Avoid asking questions that require complex language and recall – she will often find it difficult to recall the appropriate words.

- Create opportunities to use language by looking through magazines and talking about the pictures, singing and getting Mary to finish off familiar phrases such as 'See you later…alligator' (in the right context). If she can't finish the sentence, do this for her and then repeat.

- Introduce things to talk about, such as what is happening in the garden, photos, familiar items.

- Mary is not able to predict new situations and is unable comprehend what is required of her and so can become anxious when being asked to do something such as 'going out'. Her response to something she feels unsure of will be to refuse. Provide objects of reference and visual prompts to help her to predict what is happening next, such as a towel when going for a wash, or orientation through the environment such as the dining table and place setting at meal times.

- Do not leave Mary for long periods of time in a group setting without the opportunity for close contact with carers.

- Always explain what is happening; never just move Mary without explanation.

- If Mary is becoming anxious in a particular environment, try taking her somewhere quieter.

- Avoid situations where Mary may be approached by others who are unable to explain their behaviours and are unpredictable – for example, sitting too close, removing something from her without explanation.

- Mary's use and understanding of language will fluctuate. She is at her best when she has had enough sleep and is feeling safe and comfortable, when she will have conversation and social exchanges, responding with polite conversation.

- Make sure that Mary has objects close to her – items that can be used to spark activity and conversation such as her cats or photo albums.

- Mary will communicate feelings of fear and distress through physically withdrawing, physical attack or refusal to cooperate.

- Mary is extremely apprehensive and reluctant when being supported with personal care and needs constant reassurance and explanation of what is happening. Tell Mary what is expected with hugs and a loving approach. Patience and humour often works.

- Mary needs to get to know people to trust them, so maintaining a consistent support team is important to successful support.

- Mary hates water over her head, and her ears must always be kept dry.

- If Mary appears to have hearing problems, it usually means her ears need syringing.

- Mary wears dentures even at night and will need support to maintain oral hygiene as she has some of her own teeth, which require daily brushing.

- Mary is extremely sensitive to touch, often expressing discomfort when being moved. Be aware of clothing that can cause irritation if not fitting properly and incontinence, which causes her distress. Regularly supporting Mary to freshen up is essential.

- Mary is not independently mobile and needs two people or a hoist to transfer, changing position regularly to avoid pressure sores. An air flow mattress is required at night – see care plan for detail.

- Chat with Mary on a one-to-one basis in a quiet setting, outside of the routine support to meet primary needs. Her favourite topics are her nursing career or her family.

- Mary will become agitated when frightened or confused, getting particularly upset by intrusive intervention such as being changed or undressed, treating this almost as an assault. During these times there is a risk that she can hit out, grab clothing, resist support and throw objects.

- Always remember Mary's reactions are caused by a carer's action or interaction. They are not the result of considered logical thinking but are directly brought about by a feeling she is experiencing.

What's working and what's not working from different perspectives

What's working for Mary

- Being at home again.

- Family visiting.

- Having her own possessions around her.

- Being supported by staff whom she knows.

- Being around familiar people at the day centre.

- Watching the things she enjoys on TV.

- Watching her favourite DVDs.

- Listening to the radio at night when in bed.

- Being able to look out of her window and watch the birds and ducks.

- Lots of small snacks.

What's working for the family

- Mary is maintaining her weight.

- Gentle introduction of new team members to Mum.

- That Mum has support available 24 hours a day.

- Mary gets her own space as well as being with other people.

- Mary is no longer being banned from the day centre.

- Mary is still able to let us know how she is feeling through her behaviours and we are getting to understand more and more what she is telling us.

- Community health care funding (37 hours per week) for one-to-one support for all her physical/health needs to be met.

- Belief and desire from staff at the extra care setting that Mary can be supported in her flat and does not need a nursing home.

What's working for the staff team

- That Mary is in a structured placement during the day.

- The contact and involvement with family.

- Family managing all Mary's finances and shopping appointments.

- Family understanding of dementia and belief that people living with dementia should be supported in their own homes to lead the best possible lives.

- Mary came back from hospital and didn't go into a nursing home.

- Mary fits in with routines that work for them, such as Mary being supported to get up early by night staff before the day shift starts.

- Working flexibly with Mary. For instance, if she will not eat, leaving it and going back to try later. This also avoids confrontation with Mary.

What's not working for Mary

- Being rushed.

- Being done to, rather than sharing an experience. For example, staff helping Mary to eat see it as a task; they're not eating with her and sharing the experience. Mary will offer them some of her food and feel hurt when they refuse.

- Being woken too early.

- Lack of feeling of purpose.

- Day centre six days a week without real structure to the days there.

What's not working for the family

- Mary's resistance to food and drink.

- Pain management – Mary is not swallowing her painkillers.

- The 37 hours of community health care funding time isn't always utilised in the best way. The focus is on tasks rather than Mary's experience, which, with the right support, could be great.

- Criticism from health professionals on their calls that Mum is occasionally still in bed at 8.30am on a Sunday morning.

- Fear of malnourishment.

- Communication between the day centre and extra care home-based team – for example, sharing information with each other about what Mary has been eating and drinking. Also, Mary may come home from the day centre animated, but there is no sharing of information as to what made it such a great day.

- Rigidity of time and task. Mary's routines are dictated by the shift patterns – for example, being supported to get up between 7 and 7.30am every day.

- Staff are not always recognising Mary's behaviour as an expression of something, seeing it rather as aggression or moodiness.

- Concerns that Mary is supported to get up, have a wash and get dressed in 30 minutes. Being rushed really does not work for Mum and for this to be a good experience it needs more than 30 minutes. Time allocated for Mary to eat and drink is not being used in the most effective way to deliver a good experience.

- Those little extras we expect such as moisturiser on Mary's face, doing her hair nicely, her clothes arranged tidily, putting her jewellery on, finishing her outfit with a nice scarf are not happening. This suggests the focus is on getting the job done, as opposed to Mary's well-being. Those things that increase well-being are not happening consistently.

- Staff don't always think creatively. For instance, Mum's feet really smell sometimes and she could have a foot spa while staff are preparing her meal.

What's not working for the staff

- Mary will physically attack or refuse to cooperate when being supported with personal care.

- The constant fear that Mary will fall.

- Worry that Mary isn't eating and drinking enough.

- Poor communication between the day centre staff and extra care home-based staff.

Figure 6.5 shows some of the actions that the group developed to change what is not working and keep what is working.

Who	Will do what	By when
Jen	Buy some strawberry-flavoured liquid painkiller for Mary.	March 12th
Jen	Write up a list of behaviours that would indicate Mary is telling you she is in pain.	March 12th
Jen	Make available reading material and learning resources to influence staff's thinking.	March 20th
Team manager	Have a session with the team about moving away from a focus on tasks to shared experience, based on what we are learning is important to Mary and what best support looks like to her. Also draw their attention to the risk assessments on falls and remind staff not to de-skill Mary.	April 2nd
Jen	Talk with team manager about the idea of staff sharing a meal or having a drink with Mary while helping her to eat and drink to improve the quality of the experience and bring about the shift in culture.	March 18th
Team manager	Discuss arranging suitable times for health professionals to see Mary which work both for Mary and the district nurse.	March 18th
Jen	Speak with the service manager who manages both extra care and the day centre to explore improvement in communication – explore introduction of learning logs to share information.	March 29th
Jen	Arrange to meet Mary's key worker to explore ways that staff might pay more attention to detail when supporting Mary – for example, the foot spa, adding a nice scarf to finish off her outfit.	March 20th
Jen	Revisit with the key worker and the manager where the allocated continuing healthcare hours are and how best this time can be used to give Mary the best possible experience. For example, instead of three 30-minute blocks, leave Mary to lie in and then have a 90-minute uninterrupted time slot with her.	March 20th

Figure 6.5 Mary's action plan

Today life is very different for Mary. From somebody who looked continually vacant, flat and unalive, Mary's progress since returning to her own home has gone from strength to strength. She has begun to walk, taking a few steps at first with the support of staff, because she wanted to straighten and move some of her ornaments. Mary's family are convinced that this transformation would never have come about had she not returned to the flat she loved, with the things that mattered around her and a group of staff who were continually listening and learning from Mary, using person-centred practices to do so, and sharing and capturing what they learned.

Five months after the person-centred review above, Mary continues to require the pressure-relieving mattress and occasionally incontinence products, but she is now far less reliant on mobility equipment to transfer or get around her home, and food supplements are no longer a necessity to maintain nutrition. Being surrounded by people who give her personalised support has rekindled Mary's fighting spirit and zest for life. Her recovery would surely be seen as remarkable for any older person, but the fact of her dementia being in its later stages makes her story even more remarkable – recovery is a rarely used word where people are living with dementia. Mary's story shows how important it is to have rich information about what is important to a person and how best to support them from their perspective and to ensure that information is acted upon and kept 'live'. The person-centred review was a quick way to gather all of that information and to make sure that people were listening to and acting on what was working and not working for Mary.

This is how Jenny, Mary's daughter, described the person-centred review:

> What makes the difference is that it starts and ends with Mum. Everyone's contribution mattered and each contribution was given equal importance. It felt OK to share problems but also to work together to reach solutions. It was like an event rather than a formal review; we had fun together getting to know more about Mum. Running the review in this way gave everyone the opportunity to see my mum as a real person who has lived a full and varied life. Mum really enjoyed having people in her home with tea and cakes and she was able to contribute on her terms. She enjoyed hearing what people liked about her; I could see her physically grow with pride. I liked the way all the information was able to be used to develop a one-page profile and then added to for her person-centred care plan that is used by Mum's staff team and other professionals.

Developing a one-page profile from a person-centred review

As Jenny said, a person-centred review is a great way to get a one-page profile started. If you are taking information from a person-centred review to develop a one-page profile, keep the following things in mind (Sanderson and Lewis 2012):

- Remember to add detail. The initial information gathered will often be single words to describe what is important to and for the person. We now want to develop this into fuller thoughts, with more detail. For example, if 'whisky' was written in the 'important to' column, then this could be developed further by saying 'having a small whisky every day, especially single malts from Islay'.

- Remember to separate what is important to you from what is important to the person. If it is important to those who support the person that she takes a shower every day, but it is not important to her, then reminding her to take a shower goes under what other people need to know or do, not under what is important to her.

- Don't forget to put what needs to be absent from the person's life, what must not be an issue. For Julia, not to live next to noisy neighbours who play loud music at night was important to her (from a past, unpleasant experience).

- Remember that if someone needs a lot of help in getting things done and can't tell people how they like to have it done, you need to detail that part of their routine in such a way that someone who has never met the person could still get it right.

- Remember that if the one-page profile has information that the person does not want everyone to know, you must see if you can develop public and private one-page profiles. The private one-page profile is only available to those who need to know. Where there are issues of safety, this may not work, but where there are issues of intimate personal care, it almost always works.

The 'bottom line questions' for one-page profiles

- From reading it, does it make you feel that you know the person?

- Does it give you enough information to support the person well, even in a new situation?

- Is there a balance between detail and brevity? Is there enough detail to understand what is meant and who the person is, but not so much detail that the person-centred description will not be read?

- Is it written in everyday language that is easy to read?

Using person-centred thinking tools to address 'what is not working'

There is a range of person-centred thinking tools that can help to address what is not working for someone who needs care and support. In Joe's story we can see how the team leader thought about which person-centred thinking tools could help to change what was not working for Joe.

Joe's story

Joe lives in a residential service supporting 60 people with dementia. His wife, Angela, was increasingly worried that as his dementia progressed, she was losing touch with him. Joe had always been an outgoing man, at the heart of his community, running the Scout group for 30 years and also training youngsters to box at the local gym near his home in Bury. Joe had been a fireman before changing career and joining a well-known hotel chain, eventually working his way up to the post of chief executive. Angela says she always admired his ability to strike a good work–life balance, ensuring his family was a major part of his life while working in a high-pressure role. Their two sons, Joe Junior and Tom, went to the gym and Scouts with him and weekends were always spent doing things together as a family, from visiting the zoo to picnics, hiking, quad biking – as Angela says, 'it could be anything but Joe always made it fun'. They enjoyed a whole array of holidays – cruises, golfing holidays, adventure holidays: 'Joe was always one for encouraging us to try new things.'

Joe developed early-onset dementia eight years ago when he was 58. He no longer communicates typically, and although he does use words, it is difficult to work out what he is telling us. What was clear, however, was that Joe was unhappy much of the time. His family and the staff team wanted to find out how to support Joe to live a better life, but they felt stuck.

Val, the assistant manager at the home, arranged a person-centred review for Joe. The family and staff team looked at what was working and not working from their perspectives and made a 'best guess' at what was working and not working from Joe's perspective. They also generated a list of questions to answer and issues that needed to be resolved as part of the action planning.

Val looked at what is not working for Joe and thought about what this meant in terms of what the team needed to learn or do and which person-centred thinking tools could help with that. What she came up with is shown in Figure 6.6.

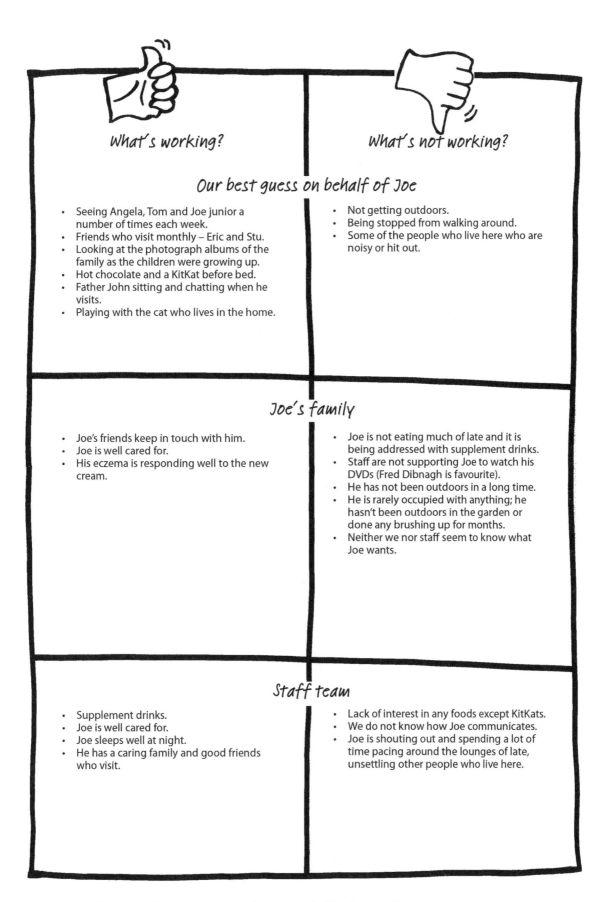

Figure 6.6 What is working and not working in Joe's life, from different perspectives

They realised the key thing that wasn't working was that Val and the staff team no longer understood how Joe was communicating with them as his ability to use words had deteriorated. They prioritised this as the first area to focus on. Val explained how the communication chart was a practical and helpful way of breaking this issue down into manageable chunks, making it much simpler for everyone. Understanding his communication was also fundamental to providing person-centred support to ensure that Joe was heard and able to participate as a full and active member of the home community, regardless of his increased support needs.

Val introduced communication charts to all those involved in Joe's life by running a session for the staff team on thinking differently about what is happening to a person (or around them), looking at and interpreting what they are doing or communicating using non-verbal signs and cues, and exploring what this means in order to support them well. The staff team could see that the communication chart was a simple but powerful way to record how someone communicates with his behaviour and how we are communicating with him. The staff started to work differently with Joe, paying attention to how he was communicating, and saw how Joe now relied heavily on non-verbal methods of communication – body language, facial expression and gestures.

Val also supported the team to use the relationship circle and life story to think about who could help them learn more about Joe's communication and whether there was information from his life story that could provide clues. Joe's wife, Angela, and his two sons, Joe junior and Tom, shared their understanding of Joe's communication. One of the key pieces of information Angela gave the team when developing his relationship circle and talking about his life story was that Joe had left the fire service some 30 years earlier after the traumatic experience of carrying four young children out of a house fire, only one whom survived. This explained what was happening within Joe when he was screaming about the burning children and grabbing out at staff. It helped them think together with Angela and Joe's consultant about how best to support him during these distressing episodes. Figure 6.7 is an extract from Joe's communication chart.

At this time	When Joe does this	We think it means	And we should
Meal times	Lays his head on the table and pushes his plate aside.	He does not like the food or he is not hungry.	Offer an alternative from foods Joe's family have said he enjoys.
Anytime	Is bright, alert, animated and shouting out, pacing around quickly.	He wants company or something to do.	If Joe still refuses it, leave it and offer him something later.
Anytime	He shouts out about children being stuck in fires and the babies are trapped.	Hallucinating – reliving the rescue of children from a house fire.	If the weather is fine, going into the garden and brushing the paths is good. Could be a good time to put on Joe's DVDs (Fred Dibnah) and enjoy them with him. Sit with him, listen to him, chat with him.

Give PRN medication – Joe usually takes this without issue. Support Joe to a quiet room, stay with him and put on a Val Doonican CD as this soothes him. Sit with him, rub his hands, sing along. |

How Joe communicates with us

Figure 6.7 Joe's communication chart

In the next chapter we look at some of the other person-centred thinking tools that can usefully supplement what we have already learned and enable people to keep reflecting, learning and acting on this information.

Chapter 7

Further Reflection, Learning and Action

Taking time to stop and think together helped us make a very different decision about Fred's care. Instead of going into a hospice for respite, support comes to Fred and I go away for a break.

Freda, Fred's wife

To ensure that people with dementia have as much choice and control in their lives as possible, and to deliver personalised services, we need to keep learning about what is important to and for the person and the balance between the two. Person-centred thinking tools help us learn about the person living with dementia and how they communicate, and capture this information on a one-page profile and communication and decision-making tools. Person-centred reviews are a way to keep this information updated and make sure it is acted upon by asking what is working and not working from different perspectives. In this chapter we describe two more person-centred thinking tools that help us reflect and learn, and add to the depth of information that we have about an individual and their life. The tools for reflection and learning are the *4 plus 1 questions* and *learning logs*.

4 plus 1 questions

Using the *4 plus 1 questions* reinforces a positive habit – that of valuing mindful observation and learning.

Michael Smull (in Stirk and Sanderson 2012)

This tool supports reflection and learning about what works and doesn't work. It can be used around a particular area of an individual's life – for example, sleeping patterns – or with a staff team around a project.

The *4 plus 1* person-centred thinking tool asks the following questions:

- What have you tried?

- What have you learned?

- What are you pleased about?

- What are you concerned about?

The answers to these questions lead to the 'plus 1' question, which is:

Based on what we know, what should we do next? (Sanderson and Lewis 2012, p.85)

The information gained through this process both generates further actions and elicits information that can be used to update the individual's one-page profile.

The *4 plus 1 questions* are an efficient way to gather what people have tried and learned and to share this and make it visible to everyone. One approach is to put up sheets of flipchart paper in a team meeting, with the four questions (What have you tried? What have you learned? What are you pleased about? What are you concerned about?), and ask people to write on them. This is a way to ensure that everyone's perspective is heard and to make sure that issues are addressed and not overlooked.

The *4 plus 1 questions* are a quick way to work out better ways of supporting people, and staff are less likely to continue to do what is on the 'what are we concerned about' list.

Fred and Freda's story

Fred and Freda have been married for 45 years; they are described as a perfect match. Fred was diagnosed with dementia in 2004. Freda and Fred made a decision to do as many of the things they had always wanted to do during the earlier days of Fred's diagnosis. They went fishing, on four cruises and, crucially for Fred, went to Wembley stadium to watch his team, Chelsea, lift the FA Cup. So Fred continued to live well and spent many happy days with Freda.

Over the last two years Fred's dementia has had a much greater impact on both partners. Fred has become totally dependent on Freda and she was finding it difficult to cope, despite having five nights' respite each month when Fred was admitted to a local hospice. This was not working for Fred, Freda or the staff team who supported Fred at the hospice. Freda describes these times as the worst part of their journey together. Although she was getting a regular break from the physical demands of caring for and supporting Fred, her emotional distress at seeing him so unhappy and unsettled at the hospice was creating so much anxiety for her that she considered the option of a residential home, although that was something neither of them wanted.

The team supporting Fred and Freda decided to use the *4 plus 1 questions* and asked Freda to share her contributions with them too. This is the information they gathered and the resulting action that they all believed would work best for Fred (Figure 7.1).

4 + 1 Questions

What have we tried?

- Used end room to avoid disruption to others.
- 1-1 support.
- Night sitting.
- Sedation.
- Expert advice – bringing in consultant from the dementia clinic. Visit from Admiral nurse.
- Male staff.
- Wife staying until Fred falls asleep at night.
- Playing music – Mozart.

What have we learned?

- 1-1 night sitting aggravated Fred further.
- If two nurses were unable to support Fred, there was no point in calling more staff in.
- Using the end room – too much activity going on because it is near the nurse station which disturbed Fred further.
- The sedation didn't work due to the knock-on effect on Fred's well-being.
- Expert advice (consultant/Admiral nurse) couldn't suggest anything further to try.
- Fred appeared to respond better to male staff.
- Freda staying until Fred fell asleep didn't help as he simply woke up distressed soon after she left.

What are we pleased about?

- Experts, i.e. consultant, Admiral Nurse said staff were doing a good job and couldn't offer any further ideas – reassuring to staff.
- Male staff having a positive impact.

What are we concerned about?

- Staff do not have specific training in dementia care.
- The facilities/environment of the building are confusing to Fred.
- Fred gets up in the night and appears to threaten others while trying to leave the hospice and that could result in harm to himself or others.
- The amount of time nurses have to spend with Fred leaves other patients unsupported.

What do we need to do next?

- Explore the sitting services from a local provider organisation, so that Fred can be supported in his own home while Freda goes to stay with her sister and gets a break from providing support this way.

Figure 7.1 4 plus 1 questions about Fred's support

The result of doing this was that instead of going to the hospice, Fred is supported at home while Freda has a break away from home and stays with her sister. This seemingly simple solution has made life much more bearable for both Fred and Freda.

The *4 plus 1 questions* are a great way to bring together the reflections of different people to enable them to come up with a way forward together, as you can see from Fred and Freda's story. In contrast, the *learning log* is a way for individual reflection on a situation.

Learning logs

Every service requires the daily recording of progress and change, although the records are called different names in different services. These notes record what has happened, but not necessarily what we have learned. Even where they do record learning, they are likely to be filed away and this learning will not be gathered, synthesised and shared with everyone supporting the individual. Amy's story illustrates this (Sanderson and Lewis 2012, p.88):

> Amy hated medical appointments. A nurse who worked with Amy recorded what happened at her medical appointment but not what she did to help Amy cope with waiting around for it. Rather than have Amy wait in the doctor's office, she took her through a drive-through car wash. Amy, who did not communicate with words, was happier and more excited in the car wash than anyone had ever seen before. The creative and skilful way that this nurse supported Amy was not part of her nursing notes, and therefore was not recorded. This story prompted the development of the learning log.

People who support people living with dementia, in whatever role, are learning important information about what matters to the person and how to support them well. The *learning log* is a process to learn about new activities or situations. Usually, this gets lost as it not expected to be recorded and this knowledge then leaves when the staff member leaves.

Learning logs are a way to record learning and reflections. Recording what works makes it more likely that the activity or event will happen again. They are most powerful when people are trying out new things – for example, Jenny going shopping (see Figure 7.2). It is vital that we are not asking busy staff to spend time writing information that will not be used. That does a disservice to the people who provide support and takes time away from the person who receives support. We need to tell and show people how their work will be used.

It is therefore important that after four or five learning logs have been completed, the manager looks at these to see what has been learned and what needs to change about how we are supporting the person. The manager then needs to use this information to update the person's one-page profile as there is likely to be learning about both what is important to the person and how best to support them (and possibly appreciations too).

Therefore the information from the learning log has to be used in the same way as the *working and not working* information is used:

- Those things that are working need to be maintained. These can be added to information on 'how best to support the person'.

- Those things that are not working need acting on to change them.

As more information is collected in the learning logs, we can look for information from them to add to the one-page profiles about what is important to the person and how best to support them. This keeps one-page profiles 'alive', not just a piece of paper that sits in a file. Learning logs are an important way to capture learning about how we are implementing the outcomes and actions from person-centred reviews.

They can be easily shared in a daily communication notebook to let family members and visitors know what the person has been doing and for family and friends to add their thoughts and knowledge of the person.

Where the same people are doing the same activity in the same circumstances over and over, the learning log will slowly lose its power and purpose. Just automatically replacing progress notes with learning logs and then not summarising and acting on this learning will breed what Michael Smull calls cynical discontent.

Jenny's story

Jenny is living with dementia and her home for the last three years has been an independent hospital in the North-West. Jenny is a retired florist and has been married to Neil for 45 years. Jenny loves his daily visits, and also seeing her daughter, Lisa, each week.

The team who support Jenny were aware she rarely moved out of the lounge in the hospital and no longer used any words to communicate. They decided to try different ways to support Jenny and to record this by using learning logs (Figure 7.2).

Each month the manager and staff team who support Jenny go through the completed learning logs to pull out what they had learned was working well, which they could build on, and what was not working, which they needed to do differently. The manager used this information to update Jenny's one-page profile about what was important to Jenny and how best to support her from her perspective. The following information came from this learning log (Figure 7.3).

Date and time	What did the person do? (what, where, when, how long, etc.)	Who was there? (names of staff, friends, others, etc.)	What did you learn about what worked well? What did the person like about the activity? What needs to stay the same?	What did you learn about what didn't work well? What did the person not like about the activity? What needs to be different?
10th November 11.00am–2.30pm	Jenny went to the Trafford Centre to go shopping for some new clothes.	Sam (a member of staff), and Joan (who lives at the hospital).	Jenny enjoyed lunch in Pizza Hut – ham and pineapple pizza. She took great interest in the plants and flowers section in Marks & Spencer.	Jenny got tired very easily when walking around. She appeared anxious when looking in the mirror at a jacket she tried on – the shop assistant was moving the mirror towards Jenny as she tried to move away from it which distressed her further. Next time go out to a garden centre for lunch.
28th November 2.00pm–3.00pm	Jenny went to a pottery class in the hospital.	Michelle (support staff), Jess the craft instructor, Tom and Nora (who live with her).	Standing at the window looking outdoors whistling when she heard the birds singing – her eyes lit up.	The pottery didn't interest Jenny but again we saw her animation/well-being increase when she heard and saw the birds singing – next time we will focus on an activity which will build on this.
6th December 11.00am–12 noon	Jenny went out into the garden.	Pat (staff member).	Jenny showed enjoyment while sweeping up the autumn leaves. She was humming and in general we feel she was engaged and content. Loved feeling the leaves in her hands, listening to the birds and rubbing her hand along the bark of the trees. Pat's knowledge of plants and their Latin names was of great benefit – Jenny seemed to listen intently.	Jenny's balance was not good – supporters to stay close without taking away her feeling of freedom and independence. Find areas where there is even ground.

Figure 7.2 Learning log about Jenny

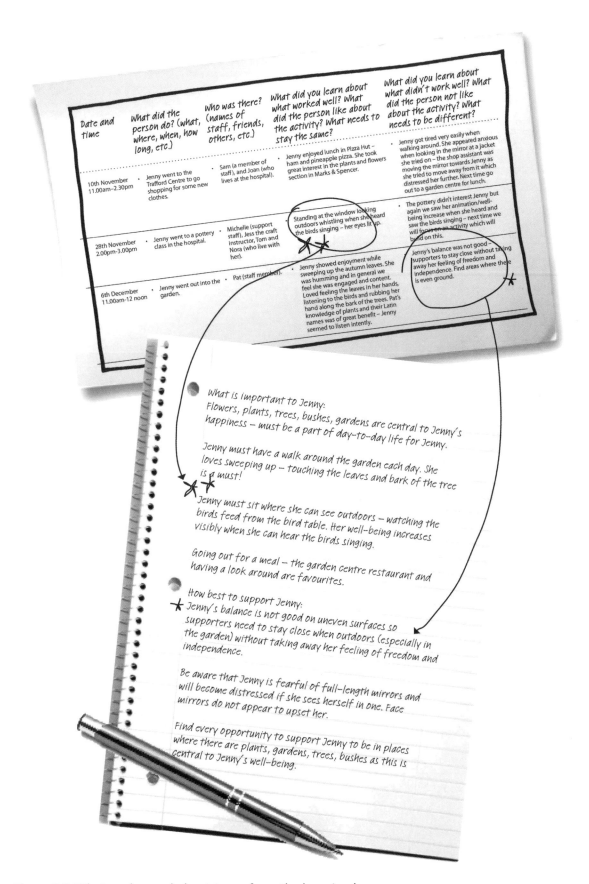

Figure 7.3 What we learned about Jenny from the learning log

In the next chapter we take a fresh look at life stories and how they can contribute further to our learning about people and how best to support them.

Chapter 8

Past and Future

Life Stories and Future Wishes

> For time and the world do not stand still. Change is the law of life. And those who look only to the past or the present are certain to miss the future.
>
> *John F. Kennedy*

> As we go through life we build up a personal history with its unique mixture of joys and pleasures, sadness and pain. Our sense of who we are is linked to that history and if we lose that history, we lose something of ourselves. For a person with dementia who is losing their memory and trying most of the time to make sense of who they are, a life story book can be an atlas, the compass, the guide to finding their self.
>
> *Tom Kitwood (Bredin and Kitwood 1992)*

> Knowledge of each person through the development of individual living stories is essential and should be seen as the fundamental step of creating relationship based care and support.
>
> *Victoria Metcalf, Dementia Consultant*

The focus on life stories has rightly been a strong theme in person-centred dementia care. It is vital that we know and understand a person's life story. As Metcalf suggests, it is fundamental in developing relationships and also helps us to learn what is meaningful to people in everyday life. Earlier in the book (Chapter 3) we discussed how learning about a person's history can help provide insights into what matters to them now and how to support them well. In this chapter, we look at how life stories not only can tell us about the past, but can help us learn about what is important now and how to support the person to enjoy a future. Little emphasis is usually given to thinking about the future with people who have dementia, other than long-term care. In this chapter we share ways to think ahead, looking at dreams and 'If I could I would…'

Life-story work is the deliberate work to enable the person with dementia to remember, share and record information about their life so far. Where the person cannot tell us themselves, family members can tell the stories behind the photos or memorabilia that people will recognise but may not recall.

There is a range of terms to describe learning about and recording the person's past – for example, life story, biography, life stories and living history. Whatever it is called, it is an important and valuable approach that has its roots in fostering and adoption work (Dementia UK 2013). Life-story work is central to both person-centred and relationship-centred care.

The benefits of life-story work are:

- It is an enjoyable activity for the person, staff and family. It will create a legacy for the family.

- It enhances self-worth and a unique identity.

- It recalls people's skills and strengths.

- It identifies past interests, likes and dislikes, which aid person-centred planning.

- It builds understanding and friendships.

- The person's well-being will be improved and so will yours!

National Institute for Health and Care Institute/Social Care Institute for Excellence (2006)

Understanding someone's history also gives an increased understanding and respect for the person, as well as a place to start a discussion or continue a conversation.

There are some excellent books and resources that cover how to do life-story work in practice (Birren and Cochran 2001; Gibson 2004; Kunz and Soltys 2007; Stokes 2010). We are not trying to replicate those; instead, we want the reader to be able to locate life-story work within the context of personalisation and person-centred practices.

Life story information, by its nature, is very personal, and there is a difference between the conversation to learn and gather information and what is recorded and how. There is a wonderful range of ways of recording this information. For example:

- commercially produced life-story book

- loose-leaf life-story book

- memory box

- audio or video recordings

- annotated photo albums

- augmented family tree

- illustrated life line

- storyboard/collage

- musical biography.

The information can come from the people themselves, as an autobiography, or supported by someone else to record their story, as a biography.

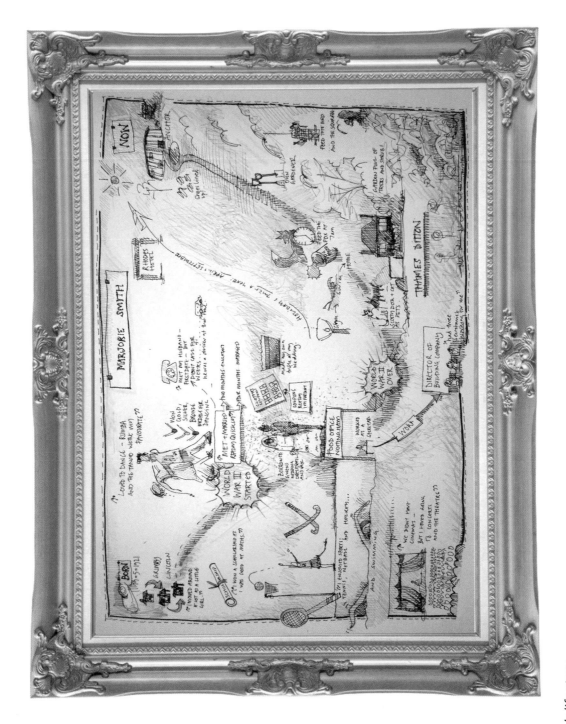

Figure 8.1 Marjorie's life story

As we said earlier, it is relatively common good practice for care homes to have a short section in their care plans about the person's life story. It is powerful when this is displayed for people to see. This makes it much more likely that staff and visitors can actually use the person's life story as a way to start or continue a conversation.

When Marjorie started to live at Swift House, she talked about her life story and this was added to her personal care file. A local artist, Paul, spent an afternoon talking with Marjorie and, as she talked, Paul drew graphics to reflect their conversation. Paul then finished the drawing, which is now framed and hanging in Marjorie's room. This is a wonderful way to start conversations with Marjorie – a 'conversational coat hanger'. A page in a personal file cannot have this effect in the same way.

Separating the past from the present and the future

As practised at the moment, life-story work typically collects information about both the person's past and what is important to them now. This information is usually kept together – in a book or memory box, or in the person's notes. We think it is important to distinguish between them, to capture life stories but to have a separate way to describe what is important to the person now and how they want to be supported, in a one-page profile. We can also learn about what people have done in the past that they may want to do again. People may remember long-lost friends with whom they want to reconnect, experiences they had and want to do again, or times in their lives that they definitely don't want to repeat and what can be done to avoid them. We can learn this from life stories, and, again, we think this is best recorded separately, and we cover a way to do this – 'If I could I would…' – later in this chapter.

Learning from life stories can also reveal a lot about what good support looks like for a person and the characteristics of the best people to offer that support.

As with other person-centred thinking tools, the information gathered through looking at histories can be added to the person's one-page profile or more detailed person-centred description by asking:

- What does this tell us is important to the person?

- What does it tell us about how to support the person well?

- What clues does it give us about the person's gifts and contributions (to add to the appreciation section)?

Table 8.1 looks at the areas that are covered in life-story work and how we can go beyond these to learn about the present and the future too, and which person-centred thinking tools we could use to record this information.

Table 8.1 Life-story questions and person-centred thinking tools

Typical life-story questions (about the past)	What else we can learn from this question about the present or the future	Where this could be recorded (person-centred thinking tool)
Where the person originated from and where they lived.	What places are important to the person now? Are there places that the person would like to revisit?	Community map If I could I would...
What has the person done at different times of their life?	What other people may appreciate and value about them. What does the person enjoy doing now? What is important to them about this? What has the person done in the past that they may like to do or try again?	One-page profile One-page profile If I could I would...
Who has been important in the person's life?	Who is in the person's life now? Who is important to the person now? Who might the person want to reconnect with from their past?	Relationship circle One-page profile If I could I would...
What has been important to them (hobbies, interests)?	What is still important to the person.	One-page profile
What they would like people to know about them.	What is important to the person. How they want to be supported now.	One-page profile One-page profile
What values have been important to them.	What other people may appreciate and value about them. What is important to the person. How they want to be supported now.	One-page profile One-page profile One-page profile
What the person makes of his life experience and may want his children, grandchildren or family to appreciate.	What other people may appreciate and value about them. What is important to them.	One-page profile One-page profile

One way to gather this information in practice is to find out what worked and what did not work for the person at different times in their life. You would not use those questions directly, but have broad conversations around them. In Table 8.2 we share some examples of the type of questions you could have conversations around (never asked directly like an interview!), covering major areas of people's lives, and what we can learn from this and where to record it.

Table 8.2 *Life-story questions and what we can learn from them*

Area of the person's history (example)	Questions	What we can learn and where we can record this
Childhood and family life	What were the very best family times? What were the worst family times?	What does this tell us about the characteristics of people in the person's childhood or family that they get on well with? **Matching** What does this tell us about what is important to the person? **One-page profile** Does this give us any clues about what good support looks like now? **One-page profile**
Schooldays	What do you remember about the very best school days? Who was there? What did you do? What about the worst school days? What were they like?	What does this tell us about the characteristics of the friends that the person gets on well with or the kind of person to avoid? **Matching** What does this tell us about what is important to the person? **One-page profile** Does this give us any clues about what good support looks like now? **One-page profile**
Favourite teachers	What kind of person were they?	What does this tell us about the characteristics of the best teachers that the person gets on well with? **Matching**

Talking about painful memories

> Remembering the way difficult times were faced in the past helps people face difficult times today.
>
> *Kunz and Soltys (2007)*

By taking this approach you are intentionally trying to discover what did not work as well as what was good in the person's past. That leads us to the question: 'Is it OK to ask people about painful memories?' One view on this is that 'remembering and sharing painful life experiences promotes greater emotional healing and acceptance of unfortunate circumstances'.

Of course this has to be done in negotiation with the person themselves, and going at their pace. You can support the person to share information that they are happy to talk about and go sensitively and gently into the conversations about what did not go well in their life. If the person gets upset, then ask them if they want to stop, but don't assume that people will always want to do that. Some people will want to be supported to talk about what was difficult and what can be learned from that. The need to put one's life into perspective becomes an increasingly important task as one ages (Kunz, Gray and Soltys 2007), but older people have fewer and fewer contacts to reminisce with as significant people die, become disabled or move into care.

You may learn about abuse in the person's past. This must be dealt with in accordance with the procedures for Safeguarding Vulnerable Adults. You will have a duty to report this to the manager, and protection will supersede confidentiality.

Learning about the past can also help us learn about what people might want to try again in the future. Earlier in the book we introduced Edie (page 31). Table 8.3 gives some information from Edie's past, shows what is important to Edie now and indicates possibilities for the future.

Table 8.3 *What was and is important to Edie and what she may want to do in future*

Important to Edie in the past	What is important to Edie now	What this tells us that Edie may want to try or do again in the future
Baking – Edie always loved to bake.	Edie's well-being is clearly increased when she sits near the kitchen hatch and watches the cook baking cakes. She has commented several times, 'It smells just like my mam's kitchen.'	See if there are opportunities for Edie to be involved in baking.
A keen knitter. Also, Edie spent many happy hours crocheting.	Edie has threatened people with the knitting needles and she has no interest in knitting any more.	Explore bobbin lacing with Edie.
She loved to walk and would walk for miles.	We have tried going out with Edie several times but on each occasion she has cried out, 'kidnap'. We know she loves to feel the wind and smell fresh air so she spends a large part of the day and evening sitting by the front doors in one of the easy chairs or in the garden if it's warm.	Sitting at the front door or out in the garden when it is warm.
Visiting Stockport market each week was a must!	Edie loves to set out tables in the home as though market stalls and is animated when rummaging through the goods.	Involve Edie in the regular car boot sales and fairs that are held in the home's grounds.
Watching Victor Mature films.	Edie is no longer interested in watching films.	
Edie's favourite pastime was reading. She was always buying books – Catherine Cookson was her favourite author.	Edie can no longer read.	Try audio books.

Thinking about the future: 'If I could I would...'

> In the context of social citizenship the idea of 'growth' is an important one, as it recognises a person's inner hopes, desires and capacity to contribute to life.
>
> *Bartlett and O'Connor (2010)*

It is not enough just to provide people living with dementia with comfort, dignity and respect; people must have opportunities to grow as well. In this section we look at hopes and wishes, and in the following chapter at opportunities to contribute.

When we have been working with staff to introduce person-centred practices, thinking about hopes, dreams and wishes has often been challenging. Staff raise concerns about how the progress of dementia means that people cannot think about a future and that their reality is rooted in their past. Staff also express concerns about 'setting people up to fail' and 'raising false expectations' that cannot be met.

The Older People's Programme and Age Concern (now Age UK) Oxfordshire ran a project where they asked people in group settings (day care centres, lunch clubs and social clubs) what they wished for and what they thought it would take to make it happen. People were keen to share and explore their own personal goals and dreams – their wishes. The facilitators then kept in touch with the club organisers afterwards to give them some support and ideas to carry this forward. There were between 15 and 20 people at each of these sessions, around 80 people in total, and they included people with dementia (for a fuller description of this work, see Bowers *et al.* 2007).

Only a few people had no wish that they wanted to share with us. Of these, two could not think of anything because:

> 'My time is full doing different things – I'm fully occupied.'

> 'My days are full with committee meetings, line dancing, bowls and Friday Club – weekends my family visit.'

But most people had two or three wishes they could think of straight away. Some people needed a bit more of a chat before thinking of something – whether with us or with another club member, the club organiser or volunteers. The wishes we were told about are grouped below under 11 general headings. Interestingly, although some wishes might well cost some money to achieve, only two people talked specifically about goods they wished they owned or could buy:

> 'I'd like a pair of amber earrings.'

> 'Find Cadbury's Old Jamaican chocolate bar, as I can't buy this in the shops any more.'

1. TRIPS, VISITS AND HOLIDAYS

- Visit a local factory to see how something (anything) is made.

- A day out or trip to (these included) Lourdes, York, London, Bath, Weymouth.

- Have a family day together.

- Go on an occasional boat trip.

- Go to the theatre in London on a Saturday night with someone.

- Have a helicopter trip.

- Go on a hot air balloon ride.

- Revisit Arizona.

- Go down a particular local walk, through a nature reserve.

- Visit the chocolate factory at Cadbury World.

- Visit a local garden centre.

- Go to Cyprus.

- Go on a world cruise.

- Visit the Eden Project.

- Revisit the Holy Land.

- Take the train from America to Canada and go through the Rockies.

- Go in a glider.

- Watch stock car racing.

- Visit one of the best and biggest hotels and watch all the top chefs at work.

- Go out in my electric scooter more, to get the courage to cross the roads. At the moment it gets used about once a year.

- Go to a horseracing event or a gymkhana.

2. DO IT AGAIN

- Ride on the back of a big motorbike.

- Try cycling again and have a cycling holiday.

- Work on a pantomime.

- Go to art classes.

3. NEW SKILLS

- Master a PC and also text messaging.

- Learn to mend punctures and generally maintain my bike (that's the downside of always having had someone to do it for me for 50 years – how I wish I had taken notice).

- Look into my family tree and find out about all my family.

4. CREATIVE ARTS

- Make a kite, then fly it.

- Take photographs of the wooden flowers I collect.

- Read more poetry and write some too.

- Read Charlotte Brontë again and share this with someone.

- Learn to paint well (paint pictures, not the walls).

- Visit the Globe Theatre and see a play there.

- Attend a concert for older people where the players do not assume that we want to listen to music from the First World War.

- Do more bead weaving.

- Write a book – it's all in my head.

- Go to a Bournemouth Symphony Orchestra concert.

- Put my life story into print, having led a most interesting one – as a policewoman during the war and then travelling all over the world with my serviceman husband. It is difficult to start, especially as I now have Parkinson's disease and find it difficult to write.

5. THINGS TO DO AT THE CLUB

- Hear a guest speaker.

6. LIVING ARRANGEMENTS

- Live with Sally (daughter).

- Join my two daughters and their families in the USA. Should I leave my friends and my British way of life to be with my American families? I wish I knew!

- Bungalow in the Lake District – country retreat.

- Have a kitten again.

7. CHURCH

- Go back to Church of England church.

- Go to church.

8. LUXURY

- Have a massage on my neck and shoulders.

- Please myself, be a lady of leisure and indulge myself.

- Personal get fit trainer, chef and chauffeur.

9. FITNESS AND HEALTH

- Learn to jive and tango.

- Walk the mountains in Wales again.

- To have good health again.

- Be able to walk about without fearing I'll fall.

- Go to classes and get really good at foxtrot, rumba, cha cha cha.

- Find out if the disabled swimming club is still operating.

- Learn to swim, without being scared of the water.

- Ramble on the Cumbrian fells.

- Walk round Farlington Marshes with someone on a [bright, sunny] day like today.

- Learn to swim.

10. PEOPLE

- Meet up with a group of people I knew 20 years ago.

- Have good neighbours and friends.

- See more of my friends.

- Talk to Patrick Moore – he's so interesting. I miss going out to the local observatory to see the sky at night

11. LIFE DREAMS

- Buy my own place.

- Have enough money to give some to charity.

- Have a lot of money to treat my family as they have been very good to me.

- Be more positive instead of not being able to make a decision.

- My dream would be to run a babywear shop.

- Go to South Africa to work with the children who are orphaned and who have Aids and are homeless.

- Win the lottery and take it abroad to work with deprived people.

There is no doubt that the facilitators did not hear every single wish held by all the older people we met, but the ones they heard were genuinely held.

Achieving the wishes

Some people, when asked, already had the contacts they needed to make their wish come true – but they weren't doing anything about it. What seemed to help them was talking to someone who was taking an interest and encouraging them. In each case, the only question we had asked to start this part of the conversation going was: 'What would you need to do to make this happen?'

Molly's story – a visit to the Philippines

A good example was a woman whose wish was to go to the Philippines with her family. She had enough savings for a flight; her Filipino daughter-in-law went every year to stay with her own family and took her children. They were always inviting Molly to go over as well, so there would be no accommodation costs. She said: 'I've been saying for ages I'll do it, but that's definite. I'm going to ring my daughter-in-law tonight and tell her, "Book the tickets straight away and count me in".'

Vera's story – a horse event

A woman who used to go to horseracing with her husband said she would like to go again. Her son had a share in a racehorse so she would ask her family if they would take her to see it race, or take her to see her granddaughter at a gymkhana.

Janet's story – a hot air balloon ride

One of the (several) people who wanted to go on a hot air balloon ride had already been on one before, organised by her son. She decided to ask him if she could go again, as: 'They're always asking me what I'd like for my birthday and Christmas, and I can never think of anything to ask for. If it's a lot of money, maybe they could all chip in, or it could be my present for both. I don't need any more talc, that's for sure!' She said it wouldn't have occurred to her to ask for something like that if we hadn't been asking the question about wishes that day.

Ron's story – discovering the Masai Mara

A man with a mild form of dementia said his wish was to go to see the Masai Mara, but he didn't think he was well enough to travel that far. Later that day, he came up with his own solution: he would like a day out at Longleat Safari Park, because his wish was to see African animals in the open.

When wishes aren't achieved

Some people may not be willing or able to achieve their wishes. One woman we met said she would love to have a massage and learn to swim, but she 'didn't have the guts'. She found ordinary life hard enough without adding something extra that she felt sure would make her more anxious. But she liked the idea of the wishes.

Another woman said she would love to get all her family together but, as this would mean 17 people, she didn't feel she would cope. She was adamant that no one was to mention this to her family, as she knew they would then sort it out but that although she loved the idea, she would hate the reality. She said she wanted it to stay as her daydream.

A third woman told an interesting variation: the minute she mentions to her daughter that she'd like to do something, it's organised for her – a trip to Dublin and an afternoon tea at a posh hotel were two recent examples. As a result, she is careful not to mention (even in passing) that there's something she'd like to do: she loves these events, but thinks her daughter does too much for her and doesn't want to add to this if she can avoid it.

> We shouldn't let the fact that something might not work out stop us trying things. Life really is like that sometimes. If it helps you, think of examples in your own life where something didn't work out – what did you do? Did you really stop trying anything ever again? Be clear whether you were the stumbling block and, if you were, either find someone else who will be able to support the person better than you did or change your approach and ask the person if you might try again. If it doesn't work but there's nothing that could have been done to make it possible, try not to write off the whole approach.
>
> *Helen Bowers (in Bowers* et al. *2007, p.67)*

Raising 'false expectations'

As we said earlier, one of the concerns about asking people living with dementia about their wishes is that: 'You shouldn't ask because if you know you can't deliver, you've given someone false hope by setting up their expectations' (Bowers *et al.* 2007, p.63). This seemed to be based on an assumption that we think we must fulfil everything if we are asking about it. So, if we ask, that's because we're going to deliver the wish. But if we won't be delivering the wish, therefore we shouldn't ask the question.

As Helen Bowers says:

> What is it about us that we come to assume that we have to fulfil everything for an older person – and so leads us to avoid asking about any aspect of life where we think we can't do this? If your friend says they want to go on a world cruise next year it's highly unlikely you'll rush out to raise the money to pay for it, organise their health jabs, pack their swimsuit, present them with the tickets and physically escort them on board. But there's every chance you'll show a great interest in their plans, ask them how arrangements are going, keep an eye out for articles and bits of information that might be of help or interest to them, ask them to send you a postcard, and then look at their photographs and home video/DVD on their return. This approach is about doing a little bit of both – a bit of practical help, and a bit of encouragement and interest. How much of each will vary from person to person, and from situation to situation. But this is not the equivalent of your paying for and sorting out every aspect of your friend's cruise. (Bowers *et al.* 2007, p.64)

Top tips from older people about achieving dreams

At two of the clubs, facilitators asked people for their 'top tips' to other older people on how to achieve their wishes. This is what they said you need when thinking about the resources to follow dreams:

- Ask your family (or whoever else buys you presents) if something could be for Christmas or a birthday or both.

- Think of an alternative that would cost less.

- Team up with others so you can share and spread the costs.

- Save up and look for discounts.

Achieving wishes in a residential care home

The stories of achieving wishes we have heard so far have come from people living at home and attending day centres and social clubs. At Bruce Lodge (a care home for 43 people living with dementia), we took a different approach to achieving wishes, as part of introducing Individual Service Funds (for a full description of Individual Service Funds and people with dementia, see Sanderson and Miller in press).

Everyone who lived at Bruce Lodge was allocated two hours a month to explore a 'wish' or do something that was important to them. There were clear parameters to this:

- People could use their two hours wherever they wanted – in the home or in the local area.

- It was on an individual basis.

- People had two hours of staff support but needed to pay for any activity themselves (staff additional costs – for example, entrance to swimming baths, cup of tea – were covered by Borough Care).

- People could choose the staff member, or the manager would match them to a staff member with shared interests/wishes, based on the staff's one-page profiles.

We phrased this as 'If I could I would…' and talked to people about this in the context of if they had some time and help, what would they want to do?

Where people could not tell us directly what they wished for, we talked with their family or other people (staff) who knew the person well. Here we acknowledged that we were making our 'best guess' about what the person might like, based on what was important to them now and what we knew about their life story. The staff member who supported the person in their two hours completed a learning log and took a photo so that we could use these to learn and reflect on our suggestion about what they might want to do.

Here is what people wanted to do with their two hours, to reflect both wishes and what was important to them:

- Ellen wanted to see the memorial plaque to the animals who were part of the war effort. Ellen at first said that she wanted to go to the park, and her son asked her if that was because of the animals. The memorial plaque was a favourite spot for Ellen.

- Annie said, 'I'd want to go back to the markets and have a fuddle (browse),' which she now does each month.

- Chrissy wanted to go swimming. Not typical for someone in her 80s! She now swims at the local pool each month.

- Jerry said that he wanted to arrest thugs and lock them up (he used to be a policeman). The closest we could get to this was to visit the police museum, which Jerry loved.

- Anna wanted to start painting again – she had been a professional artist. Since she developed dementia she had not had the opportunity to paint. A member of staff supported Anna to paint again.

What if people don't use words to communicate? Saskia has late-stage dementia, and after thinking with her and her family, our best guess was that she would enjoy going out to the park and sitting by the bowling green to have an ice cream or to have someone read aloud to her – Danielle Steele was always a favourite author. As it was a best guess, we used learning logs to check out whether this was working for Saskia and show how we could keep improving how we supported her. The learning log from going to the park with Saskia is shown in Figure 8.2.

Many people with dementia can identify and live their hopes, dreams and wishes. What holds them back is often a lack of willingness on our part to ask questions about what they'd most like to do in future. In the next chapter we look at how to enable people to be part of their communities, as contributing citizens.

Learning Log

Date and time	What did the person do? (what, where, when, how long, etc.)	Who was there? (names of staff, friends, others, etc.)	What did you learn about what worked well? What did the person like about the activity? What needs to stay the same?	What did you learn about what didn't work well? What did the person not like about the activity? What needs to be different?
10th June 11.00am–11.30am	Saskia went to the park.	Karen (staff member) and Saskia.	Dry bright day, warm but not too hot. Saskia smiled as soon as the fresh air hit her face, she hummed as I pushed her chair.	Had to come back before getting ice cream – Saskia began to groan after about 10 minutes – her arm was becoming red as it was falling by her side and rubbing against the chair when moving. Need to ask OT to provide extra cushioning for comfort before we go out again.
29th June 10.30am –11.15am	Saskia went to the park and had an ice cream tub.	Karen and Saskia.	Warm day. The cushioning for Saskia's chair protected her arm and she was comfy. Saskia hummed again and seemed to tilt her head and really listen to birds singing. Saskia seemed to focus on watching children playing with a ball; her head was moving from side to side as she followed the ball.	The ice cream made Saskia jump – too cold! Try a fruit smoothie drink next time. The café owner brought Saskia a piece of cake but she has her food puréed, Saskia shouted out and swore when it was taken away. Need to chat with the café owner and share Saskia's one-page profile. Saskia froze when a dog came near us – avoid dogs next time! Crown green bowling club play match games every Monday – go on a Monday next time.

Figure 8.2 Learning log about supporting Saskia

Chapter 9
Being Part of the Community

A Social Citizenship approach involves seeking the active participation by people with dementia in their own lives and society at large, and must be maximised and valued.

(Bartlett and O'Connor 2010, p.70)

Creating a climate where participation of people with dementia is maximised and valued is a societal responsibility.

Prime Minister's Challenge on Dementia (Department of Health 2012, p.73)

The Prime Minister's *Challenge on Dementia* stresses the importance of people with dementia being contributing members of their communities and creating dementia-friendly communities to help to achieve this. Thinking about histories and hopes and dreams can help us learn more about the person and their potential contributions. Being part of a community and having a sense of belonging are very important. 'I have a sense of belonging and of being a valued part of family, community and civic life' is the sixth statement in the National Dementia Declaration (www.dementiaaction.org.uk).

There are three person-centred thinking tools that particularly help us to think about how we can support someone to be part of their community. The first is a *community map*, the second is called *presence to contribution*, and the third is going back to *relationship circles* (see Chapter 3).

Community mapping

A community can be a neighbourhood and it can mean the people, places and associations to which we are connected. One way to learn about communities, and to think about how we can support people living with dementia to be connected, is through community mapping. Many of the ideas about community mapping were originally developed by John McKnight (1996).

When we think about mapping a neighbourhood, we can gather information about:

- physical features such as parks

- organisations

- people (natural 'bridge-builders')

- opportunities for which people would travel further

- characteristics of the local community. This could include 'third places' – those places in a community where locals gather to chat and be together such as cafés, pubs, leisure centres and post offices (McKnight 1996, p.80).

Community mapping starts with a clear purpose. Do you want to record where the person is going already so that you can think more about how to make connections there (perhaps using *presence to contribution*)? Or are you using your map to spot possibilities and opportunities to find new places where the person can build connections and contributions? Rather than collecting information about everything in a community, we start with the person's interests and use these to direct the detective work of community mapping. The best way to develop the map is, of course, with the person themselves wherever possible. This could be with their family, their staff or a circle of support.

John's family and the staff who support John used community mapping to find places where John could follow his interests. John was diagnosed with vascular dementia some years ago and his wife, Jane, and daughter, Gemma, supported him at home in the earlier stages of his illness. However, as planned and agreed between the three of them, as John's day-to-day needs increased he moved into a residential service where he is supported along with 30 other people who live with dementia. At this stage John no longer communicated with words. (You can read more about John's story in Chapter 10.)

The purpose of developing a community map with John was to support him to find hobbies and interests in his community. John's one-page profile records that it is important to him to go 'out and about' and that he loves walking in the garden, fresh flowers, black coffee with biscuits every day, and hot chocolate. John's family and staff decided to explore local places that John might be interested in.

They created a community map of a six-mile radius around the home, looking for opportunities and places that reflected what was important to John, or places that he might be interested in visiting. They decided to try:

- the local garden centre – as walking in the garden and flowers are important to John

- the engineering museum – John had run an engineering business

- coffee in the local café – perhaps John could enjoy his black coffee and biscuits here and become a regular?

Jane, Gemma and the staff drew up a plan for four months to support John to go to these three places, and used learning logs for each visit to reflect on how this had gone.

USING A COMMUNITY MAP TO LEAD TO CONNECTIONS

Once you know what the person is interested in, and what is available in the local community, the next step is to start making connections. There are different ways of making connections – for example:

- connecting people through being at the same place in the community

- connecting people by joining clubs and associations.

Figure 9.1 shows a community map, developed by the team, of potential opportunities for John to be involved with the communtiy.

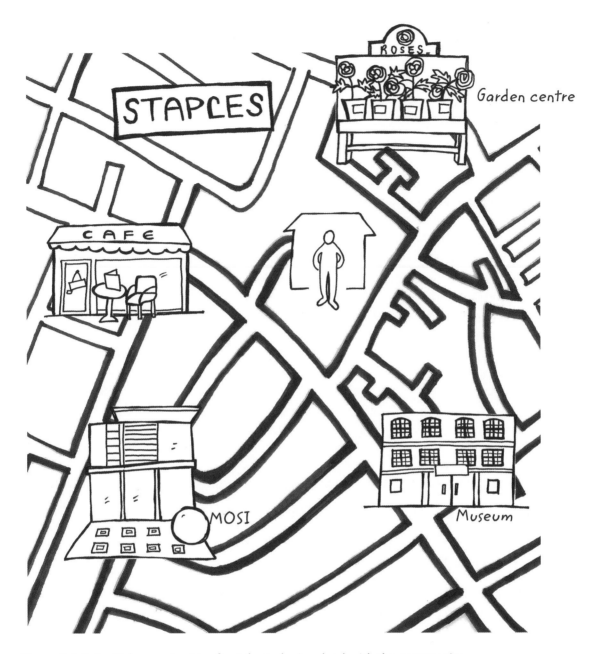

Figure 9.1 Potential opportunities for John to be involved with the community

At another care home, the manager, Jean, took a different approach to see where connections could be possible. Everyone had a one-page profile and Jean noticed that seven people said their faith was important to them. For five people this was the Catholic faith, for someone else it was the Church of England, and another person was a Jehovah's Witness. Jean and one of the seniors, Lyn, created a community map of all the churches and kingdom halls within a ten-mile radius of the home. On the map they put the names of people they knew who were connected to each church or kingdom hall. This included the minister and witnesses in these places and also staff members or family members of the people who lived there who attended. From this Jean and Lyn identified the two churches and one kingdom hall where they had the most connections. They made an appointment to see the minister or a witness for each, to ask the question: 'What could we do together to enable people to be connected to your church/kingdom hall?'

At the kingdom hall it was agreed that one of the witnesses would come to the home to meet Beryl, who had been a Jehovah's Witness all her life, to study Watchtower Society literature and the Bible, with a view to them going to meetings together at the local kingdom hall once they had got to know each other well.

A staff member who was part of the local church community offered to run a session singing hymns and reading the Bible with Paul, a missionary who will come to the home with her, with a view to Paul supporting somebody to go to church to worship with him. Paul will develop his one-page profile so the home can match him with somebody suitable who lives there.

Jean also placed adverts in the church newsletters asking for volunteers with an interest in supporting people living in the home to become involved in the church community, not just to attend services but also social activities such as coffee mornings, flower arranging, jumble sales and the like.

As well as geographic communities and communities of interest (people sharing the same faith, for example), there are also 'virtual communities' where people share an interest but may not physically meet together, connecting instead through social media. These are also opportunities for connection and contribution.

Ellen was interested in animals that served in the war. Here is a list of ways that Ellen could connect with people who share her interest:

- Leaving comments on the blog of someone who writes about cemeteries of animals (found on blogspot).

- Joining Animal Aid and wearing a purple poppy to commemorate animals who served in wars, and joining their membership group on the Internet.

- Joining three organisations (World Society for the Protection of Animals, Society for the Protection of Animals Abroad and The Brooke), which support working animals that have been injured or maltreated. They each have different ways of connecting both virtually and in person.

So far in this chapter we have looked at how you can find new ways to connect people through community mapping to identify places and people who share similar interests. Another approach is to look at where someone already goes in their local community and to think together how to create more opportunities to connect and contribute there.

Presence to contribution

Presence to contribution is a person-centred thinking tool that can help to look at connections and contributions. This helps people work out what it would take to go from simply turning up to an activity and being present to being fully involved and making a contribution.

Fong's story

Lorna is an Admiral nurse supporting Fong, who has dementia, and her husband Tony. Tony wants to continue to support Fong to live at home but he acknowledges that he needs some time to himself. So Fong began to attend a day centre two days each week, but this really didn't work for her and she would return home distressed. This placed Tony under even more pressure as he tried to reassure and settle her.

Lorna, familiar with person-centred thinking tools from her previous work, talked with Tony and his son David, asking them to think creatively with her about the options the community had to offer. Fong had always been a keen rambler and was described as one of the most jovial people you could wish to meet, who just loved the company of others. They thought about Fong's gifts. Her ability to connect and converse with others shone out, so they thought about situations where Fong could make her best contributions. They needed a local place that Fong would enjoy going to and also where the characteristics, social rules and roles of the group would offer options that would work for Fong and promote her inclusion. So they were thinking about something that would give Fong the opportunity to participate and contribute, as well as giving Tony a much-needed break.

Their favoured option was the local gym, which had a walking group from 10am to 12 noon on three days each week. Lorna used the *presence to contribution* person-centred thinking tool and it was a huge success. This helped Lorna and Tony think about what needed to happen to support Fong to move from just being present in the group to fully feeling part of the walking group and even making a contribution to it (Figure 9.2). Fong made new friends, and though initially David supported her, she soon became a popular member of the group with her zest for life, and David now drops her off at the gym at 9.45am to meet her friends and calls for her after lunch three days each week. It is something Fong thoroughly enjoys. She is a valued member of the group and appears to have a renewed sense of purpose and self-worth, while Tony gets chance to have some time to himself.

Activity	Being present	Having presence	Actively participating	Connecting	Contributing
Joining the walking club at the gym three times each week.	Walking alongside David following the group.	Going into the gym restaurant, buying drinks from the bar for David and herself.	Walking alongside other members in the group, joining their table and chatting with them in the restaurant afterwards.	Talking and laughing with others in the group as they walk, joining other members on their table in the restaurant for drinks and staying with them for lunch. David no longer walking – dropping his Mum off and picking her up.	Taking buns she has made for other members to enjoy after their lunch.

Presence to contribution

Figure 9.2 Presence to contribution – Fong's journey

Relationship circles

Community mapping enables us to think about the places, associations and people who may share the person's interests and create opportunities for connection and contribution. Presence to contribution helps us to focus on one of those places or opportunities and think about what it would take to support the person to connect and be a fully participating member. A third approach to connecting and community is to start with existing relationships and networks, and to use these as the basis for maintaining and strengthening relationships, or finding new opportunities to connect.

In Chapter 3 we shared Olive's relationship circle, which was developed so that she could stay connected with her networks and friends as much as possible. In the following story, Julie, a staff member who supported Dorothy, used her own relationship circle and connections to create an opportunity for Dorothy. Dorothy lives in a care home but she was known as a 'busy-body' because she loved tidying up. She would frequently take people's tea away from them before they had finished to try to tidy away. She loved children and was often sad as there were no children in her life.

Julie and another member of staff from the care home went on a community connecting course. On this they looked at how they could be resources to people, by looking at their interests and where they went, and each staff member did their own relationship circle and community map. Julie volunteered at the local primary school doing the milk and toast one morning a week. The head teacher was a friend of hers and on her relationship map.

Through the course, Julie came to realise that she could use her own connections and thought it would be a good match for Dorothy's skills and interests if she came along to the school and volunteered with her. This meant that Dorothy could help with the washing-up and spend a little time with children. Julie did this in her own time, with permission from her manager and the school. Julie said it was a pleasure to see Dorothy's skills being used where they were valued, instead of them being seen as irritating, and her joy in being around children was evident.

Circles of support

While relationship circles are a person-centred thinking tool to map the people in someone's life, *circles of support* bring people together to support someone to take action. A circle is simply a group of people who come together regularly with a common purpose, who think and talk together, then agree and take actions that will further that purpose.

When a circle is built around a person with dementia, the circle's focus can be to develop positive roles and relationships for the person and support them to live the kind of life that makes most sense to them. The circle can link the person up with others, but it also links everyone involved with each other (Neill and Sanderson in press).

Most people build their own circles quite naturally and informally. However, one issue that is common to many people who have long-standing disabilities such as dementia is that they become socially isolated. Often people find that the only people consistently in their lives are close family or paid carers. Here it becomes necessary to consciously build circles and connections with the person, because for some people connection does not occur easily or automatically.

Sometimes a circle can begin with just the person with dementia and one other person who makes a commitment to work to build a circle of support around the person, however difficult that is and however long it takes. In this way, circles can benefit people living with dementia who have no family or are no longer connected to their family. This more 'intentional' work of building connections in order to overcome a person's social isolation is what is meant by a *circle of support*.

Circles benefit the person, the people who participate in the circle and the wider community, but this does not mean that building circles is automatic, easy or cheap. Our experience is that both developing and sustaining circles so that they become enduring require persistence, and that the people who do this work also require support and resources. Community Circles is an initiative that is looking at what it takes to create circles at scale around people living with dementia.

William's circle of support

William is in his 70s and he and his wife, Ann, moved to Dorset two years ago. William and Ann are very sociable people, but because of William's memory problems, he has found it very difficult to meet people and make new friends, and he strongly feels the need for 'a mate'. They were referred to a circles project for people with dementia and two people joined the circle to support William and Ann – Alison, from the project, and Gordon, the memory adviser supporting William. The circle decided that their focus would be to help William to make new friends and to help Ann find information she needs to support William.

As a result of the circle's thinking, William and Ann have been introduced to another couple involved in the project and the four of them are now meeting monthly. A possible befriender has been found for William and he has also been introduced to a football reminiscence project. In time, it is hoped these new relationships will give William companionship and new links to the community, while Ann is benefiting by finding out about services that will help them in the future.

Chapter 10
Putting It All Together

John's Story

Throughout the book you have been introduced to different people who are living with dementia and seen how person-centred practices can be used to deliver personalisation. We wanted to end the book by sharing John's story. This will help you to see how different person-centred thinking tools can be used together, to listen to and support someone well, and to ensure that the service they receive is as personalised as possible, even when the person cannot tell you directly.

John's story

John is a very independent man. He owned a successful engineering business in Leicester and travelled extensively to the USA, Australia, New Zealand, Scandinavia and Thailand. He loved golfing holidays. As a boy, he supported Huddersfield Town Football Club and, as an adult, Manchester United. John was a very confident man who would chat with a roomful of strangers easily. He enjoyed socialising with friends and enjoyed a drink in his local most days.

John has been married to Jane for 44 years, though Jane says he 'never remembered the wedding anniversary!' Jane also says he is 'definitely not domesticated' as he did not enjoy DIY in any form! John adores Jane and their daughter, Gemma.

John was diagnosed with vascular dementia a few years ago. Jane and Gemma supported John in the earlier stages of his illness but, as planned and agreed between the three of them, he moved into a residential service as his day-to-day needs increased. There he is supported along with 30 other people who live with dementia.

The staff at the care home were good at making sure everyone who lives there was healthy, safe and well cared for. The information that they needed for this was clearly stated in each person's care file. However, staff found it very hard to get to know John as an individual. His speech was limited and hard to follow when he moved into the care home, and staff were unsure what John could do during the day.

'This was where the one-page profile came into its own,' said Leslie, the manager. She supported John's key worker to work with the family and the other staff to find different ways to learn about John as a person. They started with his life story and then looked at his good days and bad days, to begin to learn about what was important to John and begin his one-page profile.

They started by listening to John's life story from his family. Staff learned about what had mattered to him in the past: his love for the outdoors, art, travel and his office from which he ran his engineering business. Staff were impressed by John's business achievements and the extent of his travels around the world. This helped staff to build their regard and respect for John.

Then Leslie helped staff to think about what a good day was like for John and what a bad day was like. What they learned is shown in Figure 10.1.

Good day	Bad day
• Weather is fine and sunny and he gets to walk around and sit in the garden all day.	• People do not talk to him or listen and laugh with him when he approaches them.
• Jane and Gemma visit.	• Can't find his bedroom.
• It is quiet in the home.	• He is very sleepy.
• Lots of people having the time to talk and listen to him.	• Spending too much time alone.
• Sorting out the office, putting papers in the envelopes, creating piles of letters for posting and rearranging all the files.	• Having hallucinations.
	• He doesn't know anybody around him.
• Feeling relaxed and listening to music in his room.	• Feeling anxious about everything.
• Going out and about – the paper shop, post office, anywhere with a supporter he feels good with.	• Someone gets angry with him when he is chatting with them.
• Enjoying plenty of chocolate and biscuits and drinking black coffee.	

Figure 10.1 John's good days and bad days

From the information from his good and bad days, together with his life story, the staff began to put together John's one-page profile. This grew and evolved over a few weeks, and Jane and Gemma contributed their knowledge and expertise in supporting John (Figure 10.2).

John's one-page profile

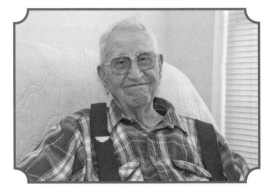

What people appreciate about John

· Kindest heart I know.
· Gentle.
· Brave.

What is important to John

· Jane, his wife, and daughter, Gemma, are the most important people in John's life; his eyes light up when they visit.
· To have space, to be in quiet areas when he is disturbed by noise going on around him. John's bedroom is somewhere that he really appears to relax in, especially when listening to his varied music collection and Jane, Gemma or a staff member sit with him and listen to him if he feels like talking.
· John doesn't do small talk and appreciates sitting without talking, unless he has something to tell you.
· A drink of black coffee with two sugars – no milk. Also orange juice is good.
· Hot chocolate and a crumpet or sandwich at suppertime are favourites.
· John must have hot milk on his cereal and sugar. He eats his cereal with a teaspoon.
· Chocolate and biscuits every day – he has a real sweet tooth.
· To go into the office and sort everything out in there and have a look around.
· To be smart and well groomed. John has his hair cut regularly with a short fringe.
· John always wears a vest and cardigan – he will insist on it whatever the weather.
· That windows are closed.
· John cannot stand cushions!
· Having a wet shave with shaving gel, not foam.
· Not to be in a noisy environment – it really matters to him to be in quiet surroundings.
· John loves going out and about. Buying office equipment for his vast offices, the pub and golf were always favourites.
· Walking in the garden – he loves fresh flowers.

How best to support John

· Always listen well to John when he is telling you something. Although his conversation may be a string of words that make little sense to us, John will feel disrespected and become annoyed if you do not give him good attention. If John offers his hand, take it – see communication chart.
· John enjoys quiet, so if the lounge becomes noisy, support him to spend time in a quieter area – his bedroom or the flowerbed area of the garden are usually favourites.
· John detests windows being open and will go around closing them.
· Offer John a tissue to wipe his mouth when necessary – he may need support to do this.
· Support John with a wet shave each morning – shaving gel, not foam.
· If John is drowsy, he is at risk of falling over if he tries to walk around, therefore staff need to support him when walking. The hoist also needs to be used if John is drowsy – see care plan for detail.
· John should be supported to sit in an easy chair when he is drowsy and should be observed due to the risk of falls – see risk assessment for detail.
· John has his food puréed when he is drowsy and staff need to support him to eat and drink at these times – see care plan for detail. He is able to eat and drink unaided when he is not drowsy.
· John occasionally will not sit at the dining-room table – staff need to offer him finger foods such as sandwiches, which he will eat as he moves around when this is the case.

Figure 10.2 John's one-page profile

The first step to personalising John's support was to make sure that what mattered to him was happening at the care home and that he was being supported consistently in the way described on his one-page profile. This is where personalising John's support really began.

As John's speech was limited, Leslie also wanted to look at how they could make sure that John was having as much choice as possible. To do this, she started a communication chart to record what they were learning about the different ways that John communicated.

The staff noticed that John found it difficult to cope with lots of people around him and the constant background noise. Jane and Gemma pointed out how much it meant to John that you took his hand if he offered it to you while talking to you or if you were talking to him – he appears to feel really disrespected if you decline. Jane found this really strange as she says John was one of the least tactile men she had ever met before the onset of his dementia – he would always shrink away from hand holding, linking or hugging in public and never with strangers! The manager suggested that they record this information in a communication chart.

John would often share funny stories, which could be difficult to follow, but what worked for John was to be listened to with enjoyment. Staff learned they should never walk away before he had finished as this created a real sense of frustration and John would shout, which frightened those around him. John's stories rarely lasted longer than a few minutes at most and then he generally walked away. This information was summarised on John's communication chart (Figure 10.3).

Leslie had started to introduce annual person-centred reviews for everyone living at the care home. Six months after they had started to use the one-page profile, there was a person-centred review with John and his family. This enabled the staff to update all the information on John's one-page profile, and to hear what everyone now thought was working and not working for John. Jane and Gemma, three of the care staff and Leslie, the manager, came to the review. They sat informally and talked about what worked and did not work. People had prepared beforehand and brought some notes. People shared their information one by one, for each of the headings in the review. Figure 10.4 shows the information that was gathered at the review about what was working and not working for John from different perspectives.

At this time	When John does this	We think it means	And we should
There is a lot of background noise	John goes very pale; you will see the colour leave his face and he hits out	We think noise causes hallucinations for John	Support John to go into a quieter area or even better out into the garden (unless the weather is very bad). He finds the flower bed area very relaxing usually. You will need to act very quickly if John goes white as he will often hit out almost immediately
Anytime	Goes very close to others, invading their space	John may want to chat with the person he has approached	If the other person is not responding to John or becoming irritated try to divert John's attention quickly – chatting to him works well
Somebody is speaking to John	Puts his hand out towards them	He wants them to hold his hand	Take the hand John is offering immediately. If it is another person who lives here and John is talking to them, quickly join them and take his hand otherwise he will become distressed very quickly.
Anytime	Pulls at his trousers	He may need to use the toilet	Support John to the toilet – see best support in the bathroom (available on a need to know basis)

How John communicates with us

Figure 10.3 John's communication chart

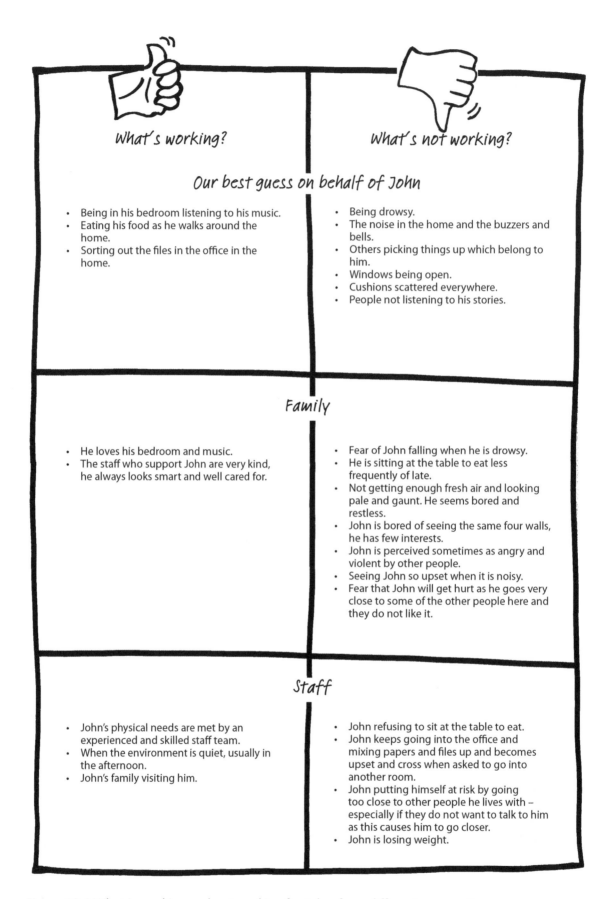

What's working?	What's not working?
Our best guess on behalf of John	
• Being in his bedroom listening to his music. • Eating his food as he walks around the home. • Sorting out the files in the office in the home.	• Being drowsy. • The noise in the home and the buzzers and bells. • Others picking things up which belong to him. • Windows being open. • Cushions scattered everywhere. • People not listening to his stories.
Family	
• He loves his bedroom and music. • The staff who support John are very kind, he always looks smart and well cared for.	• Fear of John falling when he is drowsy. • He is sitting at the table to eat less frequently of late. • Not getting enough fresh air and looking pale and gaunt. He seems bored and restless. • John is bored of seeing the same four walls, he has few interests. • John is perceived sometimes as angry and violent by other people. • Seeing John so upset when it is noisy. • Fear that John will get hurt as he goes very close to some of the other people here and they do not like it.
Staff	
• John's physical needs are met by an experienced and skilled staff team. • When the environment is quiet, usually in the afternoon. • John's family visiting him.	• John refusing to sit at the table to eat. • John keeps going into the office and mixing papers and files up and becomes upset and cross when asked to go into another room. • John putting himself at risk by going too close to other people he lives with – especially if they do not want to talk to him as this causes him to go closer. • John is losing weight.

Figure 10.4 What is working and not working for John, from different perspectives

As well as what was working and not working, as part of the person-centred review, the group thought about what might be important in the future for John (if he could, what would he do?).

If he could he would – our best guess for John

- To have an office-like environment to spend some time in, given that this appeared to be important to him and increased his well-being.

- To get out and about – for example, going to Staples (office supplies shop) or the local engineering museum.

- To go out for a walk in the local park each day.

The group looked at what they needed to do to change what was not working, how to make sure what was working kept working, and how to test out their guesses at what John might like to do in the future.

The actions included:

- Developing a community map to look at how John could get out and about more, focusing on his interests.

- Creating an office environment for John at the care home and including an office rummage box as part of this.

- Putting together a more in-depth and graphic life story to go on John's bedroom wall so that all the staff knew more about his history.

- Arranging for an appointment at the clinic for a review of his medication to reduce drowsiness.

- Making sure that all staff knew and used John's one-page profile.

John's community map

In Chapter 9 we talked about John's community map. Leslie, Jane, Gemma and the team decided to focus on the local garden centre, the engineering museum, Staples and coffee in a café, as well as walks in the local park. They decided to try these over the next four months and record how this went through using the learning log. Leslie worked on the rota so that someone was available to take John out four or five days a week to either walk in the park or follow the actions from the community map. The staff who John seemed to connect most with were Sue, Jake and Mohammed. Leslie made sure they were on the rota to support John on these visits.

Developing an office environment

At the person-centred review, the group decided to support John to go to the local Staples as a way to find out what the best possible office looked like for John – what worked best in terms of the layout – and which shelves, boxes, drawers and computer keyboard appealed to him. Staff recorded on learning logs what they learned from how John responded (Figure 10.5).

Leslie used this information to create a great office environment for John, as part of the main office area. It included two rummage boxes as part of Leslie's move to fill the care home environment with interesting material and objects for people to have a rummage in.

Learning Log

Date and time	What did the person do? (what, where, when, how long, etc.)	Who was there? (names of staff, friends, others, etc.)	What did you learn about what worked well? What did the person like about the activity? What needs to stay the same?	What did you learn about what didn't work well? What did the person not like about the activity? What needs to be different?
23rd November	John went to Staples to shop for office materials.	Pam (member of staff), Liz (volunteer) and John.	Taking the wheelchair worked! John used it when he tired, he walked to the corner of Lang Road and then sat himself in the chair. Lots of smiles from John, much happier to have the chair. Going into Staples through the small entrance avoiding mirrors. John got out of the wheelchair once we were in Staples without being asked and beamed! He walked to the office furniture and sat in an office chair. In aisle 8, which wasn't piled with stock, John spent ten minutes picking up sets of pens, envelopes and pads.	Avoid aisles 11 and 12 which are piled up really high on either side – John kept bending down really low and holding our arms very tightly. Our best guess is he feared the sides would fall in on him. John picked up some of the smaller items and put them in his mouth – avoid aisle 1 where most of the tiny items are on shelving. A dog approached us as we walked back – John looked terrified so we crossed the road and he was fine.

Figure 10.5 Learning log about John

Eight months later, the difference in John is obvious. He spends many hours in his office environment and there is a clear increase in his well-being. His wife and daughter were delighted with the difference they could see in him. He was a regular at the coffee shop and the garden centre, and had become a 'friend' of the engineering museum.

Leslie reflected three months later:

> I learned from the Dementia Congress that feeling that you matter is at the core of being a person, knowing that you matter is at the heart of being alive and seeing you matter is at the centre of carrying on in life. It feels like we have really delivered on this for John, his family and the staff who support him too, by listening differently through a set of person-centred thinking tools, the power of which is in their simplicity.

What Leslie, the staff team and the family had achieved together was developing the service around John. They made sure staff knew him well and knew exactly how to support him and communicate with him so that he has as much choice and control of his life as is possible, thinking about him in relation to being part of his community, and focusing on relationships. This is what we mean by personalisation in practice for people living with dementia.

Chapter 11

Getting Started and *Progress for Providers*

There is concern and speculation in the press about the quality of services provided in residential care home settings and the sustainability of the sector in these cash-strapped times. There is enormous pressure to ensure quality care that is safe and dignified, but also efficient and responsive to the shrinking budgets of council commissioners. Add to that mix the Government's vision for personalised services and it can be hard to know what to focus on. Personalisation is the single biggest policy issue in social care, and in this book we have shared how to move towards this on a day-to-day basis through person-centred practices.

In this final chapter we offer some ways to get started. All need a combination of energy, commitment and active involvement from the organisation's leaders, but it does not take a big investment of money, just some additional training and support, to make a significant change for people living with dementia. The best way to start, we think, is to look at the big picture and use the self-assessment tool *Progress for Providers* to see how your service is doing in delivering personalisation. Then you could either start small in one area – for example, changing the tea-time routines for everyone if you work in a care home – or make a bigger change through introducing one-page profiles and person-centred reviews for everyone (in care homes and domiciliary support).

1. Look at the big picture through using *Progress for Providers*

One way is to start by taking an honest look at all aspects of the organisation, from where it is now, to what needs to change in order to make it more person-centred and able to deliver personalisation. This big picture gives providers a basis from which they can then work out their priorities.

Progress for Providers: Checking Your Progress in Delivering Personalised Support for People Living with Dementia – Care Homes is a series of simple, practical self-assessments for providers who want to ensure they are delivering personalised services. *Progress for Providers* was developed by a group of providers, commissioners, practitioners and academics with experience in personalisation and people with dementia, working in partnership with the Alzheimer's Society. To learn more about how it was developed, please see *Progress in Personalisation for People Living with Dementia* (Adams, Routledge and Sanderson 2012), and you can find a copy of the self-assessment in the Appendix. There is also a *Progress for Providers* that covers domiciliary support and homecare, and one that addresses end-of-life support. You can find them on http://progressforproviders.org

Here are the key indicators in *Progress for Providers: Checking Your Progress in Delivering Personalised Support for People Living with Dementia – Care Homes*:

SECTION 1 – THE PERSON

1. We see and treat the person with dementia as an individual, with dignity and respect.

2. We understand the person's history.

3. We know and act on what matters to the person.

4. We know and act on what the person wants in the future (outcomes).

5. We know and respond to how the person communicates.

6. The person is supported to make choices and decisions every day.

7. We know exactly how the person wants to be supported and how to support them to be fully part of everyday life.

8. We know what is working and not working for the person, and we are changing what is not working.

9. We support people to initiate and maintain friendships and relationships.

10. We support the person to be part of their community and civic life.

11. The environment is pleasant, homely and busy.

12. We support individuals to be in the best possible physical health.

13. There is a person-centred culture of respect and warmth.

14. People have personal possessions.

15. Meal times are pleasurable, flexible, social occasions.

SECTION 2 – THE FAMILY

1. The home is a welcoming place for families.

2. Family members have good information.

3. Families contribute their knowledge and expertise.

4. We support family relationships to continue and develop.

SECTION 3 – THE STAFF AND MANAGER

1. We have knowledge, skills and understanding of person-centred practices.

2. Staff are supported individually to develop their skills in using person-centred practices.

3. Our team has a clear purpose.

4. We have an agreed way of working that reflects our values.

5. Staff know what is important to each other and how to support each other.

6. Staff know what is expected of them.

7. Staff feel that their opinions matter.

8. Staff are thoughtfully matched to people and rotas are personalised to people who are supported.

9. Recruitment and selection is person-centred.

10. We have a positive, enabling approach to risk.

11. Training and development is matched to staff.

12. Supervision is person-centred.

13. Staff have appraisals and individual development plans.

14. Meetings are positive and productive.

The progress that a particular residential home is making towards delivering personalised support is scored against each of the above key indicators from Level 1 to 5, reflecting the ability of an organisation to offer people with dementia increased opportunity to have control of their life. Levels 1 and 2 signify that residential homes are beginning to look at and address personalisation. Levels 3 or 4 signify that residential homes are delivering person-centred care. Level 5 signifies excellence, that the home is delivering personalised support to people with dementia, including individualised funding.

Table 11.1 shows how the person-centred thinking tools that you have been reading about are reflected in *Progress for Providers*, in Section 1.

This book has shared what we have been trying and learning so far. Our learning, and this book, started with Arthur, and how having different conversations and using person-centred thinking tools enabled his family and staff to make small but very significant and positive changes in his life. In his words:

> They used to leave a butty in the fridge for lunch. I hate butties. Anyway, I get a nice bit of soup or a hot pot now, something warm you know, you can't beat it. It is tons better now, they sit and have a cuppa while I eat my meals – it was miserable eating on your own, day in, day out, you know.

Table 11.1 Person-centred thinking tools and Section 1 of Progress for Providers

Section 1 – The person	The person-centred thinking tools and practices that help deliver this
1. We see and treat the person with dementia as an individual, with dignity and respect.	One-page profiles Communication charts Decision-making agreements
2. We understand the person's history.	Life-story work
3. We know and act on what matters to the person.	Good day/bad day Relationship circle One-page profile Person-centred review
4. We know and act on what the person wants in the future (outcomes).	If I could I would… Person-centred review
5. We know and respond to how the person communicates.	Communication chart
6. The person is supported to make choices and decisions every day.	Decision-making agreement
7. We know exactly how the person wants to be supported and how to support them to be fully part of everyday life.	One-page profile
8. We know what is working and not working for the person, and we are changing what is not working.	Working/not working Person-centred review
9. We support people to initiate and maintain friendships and relationships.	Relationship circle Presence to contribution
10. We support the person to be part of their community and civic life.	Community map Presence to contribution

It takes about 40 minutes to complete *Progress for Providers*. The self-assessment can be used:

- by practitioners for individual self-reflection

- with managers, to agree goals

- with the staff team to agree team and individual goals

- with other managers – for example, as a practice group, or as part of an organisational development programme.

Progress for Providers is a way to get a baseline of where you are now, so that you can make decisions about where to start to develop services further and to deliver personalisation.

2. Start small and focus on the specific

Through using *Progress for Providers* you can decide where to invest to make a difference. One approach is to then take a detailed look at one area that you want to make more personalised.

One small residential care home decided to use the person-centred thinking tool *working/not working* to look at the evening routine because the owners felt it was not person-centred. In this instance, the tea trolley came along at 4pm, with the tea already brewed in a pot and one type of biscuit for everyone. Using *working/not working* with each person clearly showed that this routine was not working for most of the people who lived there. Now tea-time is whenever people want it, rather than when it suits staff rotas. People can choose how they take their tea, and there is a selection of biscuits. Winnie, who used to be unhappy with the old system, is delighted that she can now have a Wagon Wheel and a nip of whisky in her tea.

Once you have tackled one aspect of your service, you can move on to another, and by tackling it in bite-size chunks the transformation challenge will feel more manageable. You can either start with a period of time or take each individual through the *working/not working* tool and ask them, 'If there was one thing you could change, what would it be?'

Following this change in the tea-time routine, this particular care home decided to focus on what was and was not working at night-time. They discovered that one person was distressed by having her bedroom door shut at night, because she felt reassured when she could see down the corridor by looking through the mirror on her wardrobe. But it was a fire door and night staff felt they had to close it. So, the owners fitted a magnetic smoke detector to the door, which meant the resident was safe, while her door could stay open.

You may be worried that personalising services will be a costly exercise, but it need not be; the costs of making those changes at tea-time were negligible, while the magnetic smoke detector cost £200. It is the little things that make a big difference to giving people choice and control over how they live their lives.

3. Invest in person-centred reviews and one-page profiles for everyone

Another option for developing services to become more personalised is to introduce person-centred reviews and one-page profiles for each individual. Already, in one local authority, the commissioners expect everyone in a care home to have a one-page profile.

As all commissioned services also have to be reviewed, if that review is a person-centred one, then it automatically makes it a straightforward way for a provider to find out what they are doing right and how they can improve. A person-centred review will also generate enough information for a one-page profile.

This information can also be used in *Working Together for Change* to learn about the priorities for change from the perspective of the people using the service (Department of Health 2009).

Conclusion

Personalising services for people with dementia, and enabling people to have as much choice and control in their lives as possible, builds on the person-centred care and also requires us to think differently about dementia.

We see dementia as a journey, and we are also on a journey to explore how we can change and develop our own practices to continually focus on the importance of relationships, active citizenship and community membership.

Progress for Providers

How to use the tool

The self-assessment tool asks you to look at the practices, policies, knowledge and skills of you and your staff team and at the experience of the person with dementia and their family. It takes about 40 minutes to complete the self-assessment.

Each topic enables you to score yourself on a scale of 1 to 5:

- If you tick boxes 1 or 2 you are starting to look at and act on the topic.

- Tick 3 or 4 if you are delivering person-centred care in that area.

- Tick 5 if you are delivering truly personalised services and using person-centred practices in that area (including individualised funding).

✓

Section 1

THE PERSON

1 We see and treat the person with dementia as an individual, with dignity and respect

		Tick one box ✓
1	We have only very basic information about the person and their needs. Staff struggle to describe the person in a positive way.	
2	We see the person as an individual as much as possible, but we only have information about their care needs. Most of the time people are talked about respectfully.	
3	We see the person as an individual with strengths and qualities. People are consistently described and treated with dignity and respect.	
4	Staff describe people positively. We have recorded information about the qualities and strengths of each person we support. We don't just record this, we try to use it in our day-to-day support and in our conversations with the person. Dignity is seen as everyone's business and every staff member sees themselves as a 'Dignity Champion'.	
5	We know and have a record of each person's gifts and qualities. We use a variety of ways to communicate how we value each person. We use the information about what we value about individuals in their day-to-day support. People are described and treated respectfully and positively, as individuals, by all staff. Staff feel comfortable expressing positive feelings to people.	

2 We understand the person's life history

		Tick one box ✓
1	The only information that we have about the person is in the care plan. Any record of their life history is likely to be in the context of negative experiences or behaviour.	
2	We know it is important to know about the person's life history but we don't have time to do this.	
3	We are committed to finding out about each person's life history and have started to work with a few people to write their histories when we have time.	

4	We have recorded histories for most of the people we support. We have different ways to record and share people's history, according to what the person wants. We are starting to use this information in our conversations with people. We have a plan to complete histories for everyone.	
5	We know and have a record of each individual's personal history. This is recorded in a way that works for the person, (for example, on a history map, life-story book, timeline, scrapbook, memory box or DVD). We use this information in our day-to-day conversations and support. We share ourselves through our own life stories.	

3 We know and act on what matters to the person

		Tick one box ✓
1	We focus on keeping people clean, fed and safe. We do not know what matters to each person. Our priority is to look after them.	
2	We know we need to recognise what is important to people, but we don't have the time to do this. We make sure that staff use the individual's preferred name.	
3	We have started to find out about and record what is important to the person, and we are using person-centred thinking tools to help us do this (for example, *good days and bad days*, *relationship circles*, learning about people's routines). This information is starting to change how we support people.	
4	Most people have a record of what matters to them (for example, a *one-page profile*). Staff use this information in conversations and how they support people. New staff use this to get to know the person quickly.	
5	We know what is important to each person we support. This is clearly recorded and includes specific detailed information, including relationships, sexuality, routines, interests and ways of participating. Every person has a *one-page profile*. Staff intentionally work to make sure that what is important to the person is happening purposefully in their day-to-day life. Where there are obstacles to achieving this, these are shared with the managers, who help to find ways around this.	

✓

4 We know and act on what the person wants in the future (outcomes)

		Tick one box ✓
1	Our job means focusing on the here and now.	
2	We think it would be good to plan for the future but we are not sure if it is our role and we don't have the time to do this.	
3	We are trying to help some people think about their future and what we may need to do to help with this.	
4	We help everyone think about their future; what they may like to try or do. We have a record of this and actions that we are working on. This includes advance decision-making about end of life care and arrangements.	
5	We know what people want in the future; their dreams, hopes and aspirations. We have gathered this information from the person and those who know, love and care about them. There are specific, measureable, achievable and timely actions for us, to help people to achieve their wishes (outcomes). We are clear about our role in this and how to support the person to make changes themselves. We review progress with the person. We have person-centred advance decision making in place for end of life care and arrangements (for example, using *Living Well: Thinking and Planning for the End of Your Life*).	

5 We know and respond to how the person communicates

		Tick one box ✓
1	We support people by following our policies and procedures; we do not specifically record how people communicate.	
2	We realise that we need to understand more about how people communicate and what they are trying to tell us.	
3	We have started to introduce communication charts as a first step. Staff are now beginning to understand that all behaviour (including 'challenging behaviour') is communication and are developing their skills in observing, recording and communicating with people.	
4	We use communication charts with the majority of the people we support. Staff understand their own role in effective listening and communication and know how to respond to people.	

5	We know and respond to how the person communicates. This is clearly recorded (for example, using communication charts) and staff know what a person means when they behave in certain ways and how staff should respond. These are up to date and used consistently by all staff.	

6 The person is supported to make choices and decisions every day

		Tick one box ✓
1	The people we support are not involved in decisions about their life.	
2	We realise that people should be involved and included in any decisions about their life. We also recognise that this could help people feel more in control. We do not know how to do this yet. We use best interest meetings.	
3	We have started to develop decision-making agreements with people and tried out different approaches to help people to make decisions. We are using best interest meetings and engaging families to assist in the process.	
4	The use of decision-making agreements is common and we have many examples of people making decisions about what is important to them. We are struggling to ensure that this includes people with capacity or communication issues. Staff support people to record their decisions. We use advocacy from others where necessary. We support individuals to plan in advance for the end of their life in a sensitive way (for example, using *Living Well: Thinking and Planning for the End of Your Life*)	
5	Staff know the decisions that are important to the person, how to support the person with these decisions and how the final decision is made. This is recorded (for example, in a decision-making agreement). We make sure people get representation if they need it. We have supported some people to make decisions that we don't agree with and manage the tension in this. We support people to extend the range and importance of the decisions that they make, to have more control over their life, through advocates if necessary. Everyone is sensitively supported to think about and plan for the end of their life, and these decisions are recorded and shared with the family and GP where appropriate.	

✓

7 We know exactly how the person wants to be supported and how to support them to be fully part of everyday life

		Tick one box ✓
1	We have established policies and procedures for how we support people and we support everyone in the same way.	
2	We know that to support people effectively, we need to find out how they would like to be supported. We are unsure how to do this and record the information. Currently, our approach is not flexible enough to allow this to happen. We are task orientated rather than people orientated but we want to change this.	
3	We acknowledge the importance of finding out from people what good support looks like for them individually and we have begun to explore this with them. We have developed a plan to gather this information for everyone, using person-centred thinking tools.	
4	Everyone in the team is clear about what good support looks like for each person they support. We have started to record this (for example, in one-page profiles). Staff understand what this means for their practice on a day-to-day basis and are using this information to inform how they support people.	
5	We know and act on how the person wants to be supported. This is clearly recorded, is detailed, is specific to the person and staff use this to deliver individual support. The information includes the support people want in their routines, in relationships and interests, and how to help people to be healthy, safe and participating fully in everyday life. This includes support specific to the person's culture, gender, race, religion, belief and sexuality. We review staff performance on their ability to provide support in the way that someone wants. We use technology and assistive technology to get our support right for the person. People are as active in their own care as possible.	

8 We know what is working and not working for the person, and we are changing what is not working

		Tick one box ✓
1	We do not know what is *working or not working* for the people we support.	
2	We want to learn what people think is *working and not working* in their lives. We are not sure how to do this and are fearful that we will not be able to respond and make the changes they want.	

3	We have started to routinely ask people what is *working and not working* from their perspective about their life and the service they receive (for example, as part of a person-centred review).	
4	Staff are confident in supporting people to tell us what is *working and not working*. This happens for everyone at least once a year. There is an action plan developed from this. We have created a system that will gather this information from people so that we can plan strategically what needs to happen in the service.	
5	We have a process to learn what is *working and not working* for the person, from their perspective. We have actions (with a date and a named person responsible) to change what is not working. The actions are regularly reviewed with all key people, including the person.	

9 We support people to initiate and maintain friendships and relationships (For family relationships see Section 2, page 150)

		Tick one box ✓
1	The only people in the person's life are paid staff. We don't see it as our responsibility to support people's other relationships.	
2	We realise that people might want to meet and make more friends but we are fearful that this could expose people to harm and risk, and we are not prepared to accept responsibility for this. We are not sure how we would begin to find out who is (or could be) important in the person's life.	
3	We have started to work out how we can support people to build and maintain relationships. We are still worried about the risk and how to manage this. We have started to understand what is in the local community and we are developing *relationship circles*. Staff are putting a greater focus on people's interests and friendships.	
4	We have tried a number of approaches to support people with their friendships and relationships. We know who is already important in the person's life (for example, by using a *relationship circle*) and people now have opportunities to meet new people who are not paid to be with them. We are gathering the learning and sharing good practice.	
5	We support people to maintain relationships that are important to them (including sexual relationships). We support people to make new relationships with people in their home and with their wider community. We have a culture that creates positive, mutual, valued relationships between staff and people with dementia.	

✓

10 We support the person to be part of their community and civic life

		Tick one box ✓
1	It is not our job to connect people to the community.	
2	We think it would be good if people were out and about in the community more but can't see how we can do this within our current resources.	
3	We are committed to exploring ways of people being part of their communities and civic live, and we have started thinking about how to do this with a few people we support (for example, *using community maps, recording gifts and presence to contribution*).	
4	We support some people to go out and be part of their community, and we use person-centred thinking tools in the way that we approach this.	
5	We support people to be involved in their community and civic life. We use *community maps* that show the places that are important to the person and we actively support people to be part of their community and make a contribution in whatever way works for them.	

11 The environment is pleasant, homely and busy

		Tick one box ✓
1	The home looks and feels rather sterile and we don't have the time or resources to make it homely. People rarely engage in purposeful activity. It is not easy for people to find their way around. The chairs are all the same and are placed around the outside of the room. We don't have the resources or skills to develop an environment that supports people's independence.	
2	We understand the need to make things homely and well sign-posted and have tried some simple approaches to this. We are considering how the environment can be enhanced to support people's independence.	
3	Chairs are arranged to enable people to talk to each other easily. There are a few things to occupy people. People can find their way around (use of contrast, colour and appropriate signage). We have made some improvements to support independence.	

		Tick one box ✓
4	The home is comfortable and is arranged to suit people (for example, where people like to sit) and support their independence. There is a range of things for people to do. There are areas where people can sit and relax, space to do hobbies and activities, and quiet spaces. There is an outdoor space with places to sit.	
5	The environment is pleasant, homely and busy. People have as much control over their physical environment as possible, (for example, the temperature, noise levels, music). There is a wide variety of things for people to do (for example, arts and crafts, hobbies, games). There are spaces inside and outdoors for relaxation and hobbies. Staff understand the importance of how the living environment affects people.	

12 We support individuals to be in the best possible physical health

		Tick one box ✓
1	We focus on keeping people clean and comfortable. We do our best to keep track but sometimes people lose their glasses, hearing aids or dentures.	
2	We try to get people moving about when we can. We have a monitoring system that prevents pressure ulcers, falls, infections and so on.	
3	We check on a daily basis that people have the right glasses, hearing aids or dentures and try to ensure that people have regular health checks. We look out for any signs that people may be in pain. We support people to look after their appearance.	
4	We are confident that people have up to date health checks and always have their own glasses, hearing aids and dentures. We keep good records of these. When someone's behaviour changes, we look to see if there is a physical cause and look out for indications that people are in pain. We have an active programme to keep people healthy and fit through exercise programmes and healthy eating. We have a medical review that is part of their person-centred information.	
5	We pride ourselves that people are in the best possible physical health and comfort. We know and have a record of the best ways to support each person to be physically healthy, and how we will know if they are in pain. We support people to be physically active, both inside and outside the home, as part of their daily routine. We actively seek ways to reduce the amount of medication that people are on. We ensure that everyone has regular sight and hearing tests, and have a medical and dental review as part of a person-centred review. We are always looking out for signs that people may be in pain and act immediately.	

✓

13 There is a person-centred culture of respect and warmth

		Tick one box ✓
1	Staff talk over people and are focused on getting all the daily tasks done. Sometimes staff 'tell people off' and are patronising. People may be labelled (for example, 'the wanderer'). All staff wear uniforms.	
2	Staff try not to talk over people and know the importance of treating people with respect, although there is still some patronising behaviour towards people with dementia. Staff wear uniforms.	
3	No-one wears uniforms and everyone is addressed by their first name (and no separate staff toilets). Staff know the importance of developing good relationships with people with dementia and take time to talk to people as much as possible. Staff have a name badge with their first name on it.	
4	All staff work to develop good relationships with people and see this as very important in their role.	
5	Staff have a clear, recorded set of values that underpin their work and agreed ways of working in respectful, warm and positive ways. Staff are comfortable in sharing information about themselves to develop warm and trusting relationships with people they support. Staff are clear that their role is not task focused but relationship focused, valuing people with dementia.	

14 People have personal possessions

		Tick one box ✓
1	Everything is treated communally and it sometimes means that people end up wearing other people's clothes. People may not have shoes.	
2	Most clothes are labelled and we do our best to make sure people have their own clothes and wear shoes. People have a few personal possessions in their room (for example, photographs).	
3	We encourage people to have as many personal possessions as they want in their bedroom. We ensure that people have their own clothes and shoes and that these are looked after.	
4	Everyone has a range of personal possessions in their room, and we support people to take care of them.	
5	Everybody has many personal possessions and we know which possessions are important to people. We ensure people have support to look after their possessions (for example, photos, plants, jewellery, clothes, ornaments, CDs, DVDs and iPods). We actively support people to buy more possessions if they choose.	

15 Mealtimes are pleasurable, flexible, social occasions

		Tick one box ✓
1	We offer one choice of dish each meal time. We have fixed times for meals and have to work hard to make sure that everyone eats then.	
2	We have fixed times for meals, with one dish available but we accommodate dietary preferences and requirements like halal or gluten-free meals. Mealtimes feel rushed but we try and talk to people, as well as feed them.	
3	We are as flexible as we can be around mealtimes and usually offer people the choice of a couple of dishes. We help people to choose the one they want as much as possible. We try to make mealtimes sociable occasions.	
4	We support people to choose from several meal options. We pay attention to the presentation of the food so that it looks appetising. People can take as long as they want over their meals. People are encouraged to help with preparing meals or laying the table.	

		Tick one box ✓
5	Mealtimes are pleasurable, sociable occasions. People choose when, where and what they eat (for example, using picture menus) and who they want to eat with. The meals are delicious and attractively presented. People can take as much time as they want over their meals. A range of finger foods and snacks is always available. People are supported to take an active role in meal times, for example preparing meals or laying the tables. People get the support they need to eat and drink in a respectful and unobtrusive way.	

Section 2

FAMILY

1 The home is a welcoming place for families

		Tick one box ✓
1	We have visiting hours when families can come. We are strict about these. It is important that staff can get their jobs done without visitors around.	
2	We have visiting hours but we are flexible with these.	
3	Families and friends can visit when they want, within reason. The entrance is welcoming and it is easy to find your way around when you come in.	
4	We welcome family members and friends, work hard to make sure they feel at home and make them drinks when we can.	
5	Family members are welcomed at all times, including meal times. Family members feel at home and can make themselves drinks when they want. Families can meet together privately if they wish, in the person's bedroom and in other places.	

2 Family members have good information

		Tick one box ✓
1	We do not see our role as providing information for families. We answer questions that families have, when we have time.	
2	We try and help families as much as we can when they ask questions.	

3	We have leaflets and information at the home and tell families about these when they ask questions. We provide information on notice boards about what is happening in the home.	
4	We proactively make sure that families have good information about what is happening in the home and in their family member's life.	
5	Family members have all the information they need, when they want it, in everyday language. This is through a range of sources, such as newsletters, social media and one-to-one sharing. Family members know what is happening in the home generally, as well as in the life of their family member.	

3 Families contribute their knowledge and expertise

		Tick one box ✓
1	We get our information about the people we support from the files.	
2	We know that families have information about the person and we try and get this when we can.	
3	We make sure that we talk to the family and get all the information they have for our records.	
4	We work with the family to learn about the person's past as well as who they are today. We record this information in a person-centred way. We invite the family to reviews.	
5	We acknowledge the expertise of families as those who know and care most about the person. Families contribute to our understanding of the person, for example the person's history, communication preferences, knowing what matters to the person, their aspirations for the future, how they are best supported and their connection to the community. We proactively work with families to enable them to contribute to person-centred reviews (for example, by arranging them at times that suit the family) and actually providing care if they choose.	

✓

4 We support family relationships to continue and develop

		Tick one box ✓
1	It is not our role to get involved in relationships between the family and the person.	
2	We try and help families stay in touch but there is not much that we can do.	
3	We do what we can to help families stay connected, for example, by talking to the person about their family.	
4	We spend time working out how the person can stay in contact with their family and what we can do to help, for example, making sure that the person is supported to send birthday and celebration cards.	
5	We support people to remain an active part of their family, continuing with relationships and family celebrations that are important to them. We support families as circumstances and relationships develop and change. We actively work with families to share their perspective through person-centred reviews and learning what is working and not working from different perspectives.	

Section 3

STAFF AND MANAGERS

1 We have knowledge, skills and understanding of person-centred practices

		Tick one box ✓
1	None of the staff has any understanding or experience of using specific person-centred thinking tools or practices.	
2	We know that we need to develop our skills, knowledge and understanding of person-centred thinking tools but have not developed any plans to do this and are not sure how to begin.	
3	We have a plan to develop our understanding of person-centred thinking and some of the team have begun to use person-centred thinking tools and approaches. We have started to look at some of the information available on person-centred thinking (for example, the short films on person-centred thinking on YouTube).	

4	I am using person-centred thinking tools and approaches myself, and all the team know and are successfully using several of the tools. I have a *one-page profile* and so do each of the team, and we are using this in our work together.	
5	We all have our own *one-page profile* and we use this to inform our practice. We are all confident and competent in using person-centred thinking tools, using them consistently in all areas of our work to enable people with dementia to have as much choice and control as possible in their lives. Everyone can describe the person-centred thinking tools (why and how you can use them and the benefits to the person with dementia) and talk about their experience of using them, and the outcomes achieved.	

2 Staff are supported individually to develop their skills in using person-centred practices

		Tick one box ✓
1	No one in the team has a personal development plan and we are not using any process to reflect on how we work and how to develop our skills.	
2	I recognise that all staff need ongoing support and opportunities for development, to build their skills and knowledge, and a way for their progress to be monitored. I am not sure how to go about this.	
3	I have started to talk to each team member about how they are doing in using person-centred thinking tools and approaches in their work. This is on an ad hoc basis.	
4	I talk to each team member on a regular planned basis about how they are developing their skills in using person-centred thinking and approaches, and how I can support them in this. I have a record of the progress that team members are making (for example, using the *person-centred thinking rating scale*).	
5	Each staff member has a regularly reviewed individual development plan that includes how they are developing their competence in using person-centred practices with people who have dementia. This includes celebrating successes and solving difficulties. I ensure that staff members reflect on their own practice and are accountable for this. We use a range of ways to ensure each staff member has individual support in using person-centred thinking tools and approaches (for example, peer support, mentoring and person-centred thinking as a standard agenda item for supervision). We have a mechanism for recording and sharing best practice across the organisation.	

✓

3 Our team has a clear purpose

		Tick one box ✓
1	We have an organisational mission statement created by the senior manager/management team/owner. This complies with requirements. We have not considered how this should be reflected in the way we work.	
2	We think it would be helpful for the team to think about our purpose as a team but I am not sure how to go about this.	
3	We have begun to talk with staff about what our purpose is and to think about how we can record this.	
4	We are clear about our team's purpose and how this fits with the organisation's mission statement. We have developed this together as a team and with people using the service.	
5	The organisation's mission statement informs the team's purpose. Everyone understands the connection between the mission and their individual purpose and role. The team knows what their team purpose is and what we are trying to achieve together. All team members know their purpose in relation to the people they support, their team and the rest of the organisation. This is recorded (for example, in a purpose poster or team purpose statement). The team's purpose informs the work of the team and there is evidence of this in practice.	

4 We have an agreed way of working that reflects our values

		Tick one box ✓
1	We don't really think about values, we just get on with the job.	
2	We realise that we need to explore our values and beliefs as a team and how this can inform our practice.	
3	We have started to think together about our team values and how we work together. We know what is working and what needs to change.	
4	We have agreed our values and team principles and developed an action plan that addresses what needs to change, in partnership with people we support.	

5	The team has a shared set of beliefs or values that underpin their work and agreed ways of working that reflect these. These reflect working in a person-centred way to ensure that people have maximum choice and control in their lives, as part of their local community. The team principles and ways of working are clearly documented (for example, ground rules, team charter, person-centred team plan, team procedure file). The team regularly evaluates how they are doing against these agreed ways of working (for example, by using what is working and not working from different perspectives).	

5 Staff know what is important to each other and how to support each other

		Tick one box ✓
1	My team members do not know each other very well.	
2	I have started to work on ways that I can help the team know more about each other; what matters to them as people and how they can support each other at work (for example, starting with *one-page profiles* for everyone).	
3	I am learning what is important to my team and how best to support them. We are all aware of how to support each other and what is important to each other and we are working at putting this into practice.	
4	My team and I have all documented how best to support each other and what is important to each of us. We know how we make decisions as a team and the best ways to communicate together.	
5	As a team we know and act on what 'good support' means to each person. This information is recorded (for example, in a person-centred team plan). We regularly reflect on what is *working and not working* for us as a team, and what we can do about this. We have a culture where we appreciate each other's gifts and strengths and use these in our work wherever we can.	

✓

6 Staff know what is expected of them

		Tick one box ✓
1	I think each team member has a general sense of what is expected of them.	
2	All staff have a generic job description and work to organisational policies and procedures.	
3	I know that staff need to be clearer about what their important or core responsibilities are and where they can try out ideas and use their own judgement. We have started to have discussions in the team about this.	
4	Some staff are clear about what is expected of them and where they can make decisions themselves. There are still some grey areas that we need to explore more. We are using person-centred thinking tools (for example, *the doughnut*) in clarifying expectations and decision making.	
5	Staff know what is expected of them – they are clear about their core responsibilities and where they can try new ideas in their day-to-day work. Staff are clear about their role in people's lives and know what they must do in relation to the people they support and team, administrative or finance responsibilities. Staff know how to use person-centred practices to deliver their core responsibilities. Staff know where they can use their own judgement and try new ideas or approaches, and record what they are learning about what works and does not work when they use their own judgement. Roles and responsibilities are clearly recorded (for example, in *a doughnut*) and this is reflected in job descriptions.	

7 Staff feel that their opinions matter

		Tick one box ✓
1	I make all decisions; I don't involve my team. I chair team meetings and set the agenda. I set the agenda for supervision and appraisal.	
2	I recognise the need to find a way to listen to my staff team, value their opinions and engage them in decision making. I am trying to improve how I do this.	
3	My team have some involvement in setting team meeting agendas. I still make most of the decisions.	

4	I regularly meet with my team and discuss issues that they raise (in team meetings and other day-to-day opportunities). They contribute to team meetings agendas and make suggestions for supervision discussions. Some staff make suggestions for new ideas or changes. We are starting to use person-centred thinking tools to listen to each other.	
5	All staff feel that their opinions are listened to. Team members are asked for their opinions and consulted on issues that affect them. Team members feel confident in suggesting new ideas or changes to me. We regularly use person-centred thinking tools in the team to listen to each other's views and experiences (for example, *4 plus 1 questions*).	

8 Staff are thoughtfully matched to people and rotas are personalised to people who are supported

		Tick one box ✓
1	I write staff rotas based upon staff availability. The rota meets the requirements of the service. There is a system for staff and people who use the service to make requests.	
2	I have identified the preferences of people who are supported and the staff (for example, using the *matching tool* and *one-page profile*). I write the rotas and take these preferences into consideration where possible.	
3	Sometimes people who are supported are matched to staff with similar interests but service need still takes priority.	
4	My team and I know what individuals' preferences are, how they like to be supported and what is important to them. These preferences are acknowledged in the way that the rota is developed, so that we get a good match between the person and the staff who support them. Rotas are developed around people using the service, based on the support they want and the activities they want to do, and who they want to support them.	
5	Decisions about who works with whom are based on what the person supported wants. Where the senior staff make this decision, it is based on which staff get on best with different individuals, taking into account what people and individual staff members have in common (for example, a shared love of rock and roll music) as well as personality characteristics (for example, gregarious people and quieter people), necessary skills and experience. People can choose different staff for support with hobbies and interests, and personal care.	

✓

9 Recruitment and selection is person-centred

		Tick one box ✓
1	Staff are recruited to the team based on formal job descriptions that have been developed by the organisation.	
2	I know I should involve the people who receive a service in recruitment but I am not sure how to go about this.	
3	I have started to look at 'good practice' examples of ways to involve people in recruiting their support staff. We have started to explore how we can develop job descriptions that reflect what is important to the people we support.	
4	We have worked with people and identified ways for them and their families to be involved in recruitment and selection of their staff. This happens some of the time. We have developed personalised job descriptions and adverts based on what is important to the person and how they want to be supported. We use the *matching tool* in our recruitment processes.	
5	Our recruitment and selection process demonstrates a person-centred approach. We recruit people who can deliver our purpose by selecting people for their values, beliefs and characteristics, not just their experience and knowledge. Where people's funding is individualised, job descriptions are personalised to the people who are supported, using information from the *matching tool*. It is common practice for people to be involved in recruiting their staff, in a way that works for them.	

10 We have a positive, enabling approach to risk

		Tick one box ✓
1	I encourage my team to make sure people are safe and do not take risks. We adhere to all required legislation.	
2	I am aware that I need to encourage my team to become less risk averse. I am not sure how to do this.	
3	I am working with the team to help them take a responsive and person-centred approach to risk. We are starting to use this in some situations.	
4	We use a person-centred approach to risk most of the time. We involve the people, family and others in thinking this through. I ensure everything is documented and adheres to the relevant legislation.	

5	We ensure that risks are thought through in a person-centred way that reflects what is important to the person and decisions are clearly recorded. The person and their family are centrally involved in the way that we do this. We support people to take the risks that they want to take.	

11 Training and development is matched to staff

		Tick one box ✓
1	All training is based on statutory requirements. I make sure that we meet minimum legal and statutory requirements.	
2	I recognise that I need to find a way for training and development opportunities to reflect the needs of the service we provide to people, and motivate the staff.	
3	I have started to think about how I can introduce learning and development opportunities to staff that will reflect the needs of people who receive a service and also encourage and develop the team member. I have begun to look at *what is working and what is not working* for individuals and also researching what is available.	
4	We have identified all training needs, learning and development opportunities and have a plan in place. Training and development opportunities reflect the needs and wishes of people who receive a service and have been agreed with team members. Person-centred thinking and approaches are central to our approaches to training. We comply with all legal and statutory requirements.	
5	We provide development and training opportunities to all staff, including volunteers, that focus on increasing choice and control for people we support and delivering an individual, person-centred service. Within a few months of starting with the organisation, new staff have induction training that includes using person-centred thinking and approaches to deliver our purpose. Our training enables staff to be up to date with best practice in delivering choice and control for people with dementia and using person-centred practices to enable people to live the lives they want. We know that the senior staff are key to delivering a person-centred service and we have specific training and support to enable them to use a person-centred approach in all aspects of their role, and to be able to coach their staff in using person-centred thinking skills.	

✓

12 Supervision is person-centred

		Tick one box ✓
1	I set the agenda and make the arrangements for staff supervision. I meet the minimum requirement.	
2	I am aware that staff support and supervision practice needs to be reviewed. I am not sure how I can change the current arrangements.	
3	I have started to think about involving people who receive a service in staff supervision. I have talked to people and staff about how we might go about this. Most members of staff have supervision meetings.	
4	All staff (including the manager) are supervised and people who staff support usually contribute through sharing their views with me before the supervision session. Supervision results in actions and the meetings are documented. I have started to use person-centred thinking tools in supervision sessions.	
5	Each staff member and the manager has regular, planned, individual supervision. Supervision includes giving staff individual feedback on what they do well and an opportunity to reflect on their practice. Staff are coached to develop their skills in working in a person-centred way. There is a clear link between training and supervision and what people do when they are at work (for example, when people attend training, managers expect to see a difference in their work, and this is discussed in their individual supervision). The views of people supported and their families are very important in the supervision process and people are asked their views before supervision.	

13 Staff have appraisals and individual development plans

		Tick one box ✓
1	Most of my staff have an appraisal. I set the agenda and assign objectives.	
2	I have recognised that people who receive a service and their families should be given the opportunity to feed back on the support they receive from staff. I am not sure how I should go about this. Staff have an appraisal but do not really contribute to the agenda or any development plan.	

3	I have a plan in place to ensure that each member of staff receives an annual appraisal. Where possible, I try to seek the views of people who receive a service and their families.	
4	We have a variety of ways for people who receive a service and their families to contribute their views to staff appraisals. All staff are asked to reflect on what they have tried, what they have learnt, what they are pleased about and whether they have any concerns. We then agree what actions need to be taken from all the information gathered.	
5	Team members get positive feedback about their work and have annual appraisals and individual development plans. Annual appraisals include feedback from people supported and their families, about *what is working and not working* about the support they receive. This results in an individual development plan with clear goals that build on strengths, focus on working in a person-centred way, and further developing skills.	

14 Meetings are positive and productive

		Tick one box ✓
1	We have occasional team meetings but not everyone attends or contributes.	
2	There are frequent team meetings. I set the agenda and chair the meeting. There is little structure to the meeting and they are not as well attended as they could be.	
3	I schedule regular team meetings. The meeting tends to be an information-giving forum and does not often include problem solving or celebrating successes.	
4	We have regular structured team meetings, which are documented. Actions are agreed, recorded and followed up. They are well attended and most people contribute.	
5	Our team has regular, productive team meetings that are opportunities to hear everyone's views and contributions. Team meetings include sharing what is going well and problem solving (for example, practicing using person-centred thinking tools to solve problems). Outside of formal meetings, people are encouraged to use peer support (for example, practice groups and action learning sets).	

References

Adams, T., Routledge, M. and Sanderson, H. (2012) *Progress in Personalisation for People with Dementia.* Stockport: HSA Press.

Bartlett, R. and O'Connor, D. (2010) *Broadening the Dementia Debate: Towards Social Citizenship.* Bristol: Policy Press.

Birren, J. and Cochran, K. (2001) *Telling the Stories of Life through Guided Autobiography Groups.* Boston, MA: The John Hopkins University Press.

Bowers, H., Bailey, G. and Sanderson, H. (2007) *Practicalities and Possibilities: Using Person-Centred Thinking with Older People.* Stockport: HSA Press.

Bowers, H., Bailey, G., Sanderson, H., Easterbrook, L. and Macadam, A. (2007) *Plans and Practicalities: Person-Centred Thinking with Older People.* Stockport: HSA Press.

Bredin, K. and Kitwood, T. (1992) 'Towards a theory of dementia care: Personhood and well-being.' *Ageing and Society 12*, 3, 269–287.

Brooker, D. (2007) *Person-Centred Dementia Care: Making Services Better.* London: Jessica Kingsley Publishers.

Bryden, C. (2012) 'An insider's perspective on what you can do to help a person with dementia.' JKPVideos. Available at www.youtube.com/watch?v=7E49cK17qs0, accessed on 1 May 2013.

Deacon, A. and Mann, K. (1999) 'Agency, modernity and social policy.' *Journal of Social Policy 28*, 3, 413–435.

Dementia UK (2013) Available at: www.dementia.org/information-support/life-story-work/, accessed on 2 Aug 2013.

Department of Health (2007) *Putting People First.* London: Department of Health.

Department of Health (2008) *High Quality Care for All: NHS Next Stage Review Final Report.* London: Department of Health.

Department of Health (2009) *Putting People First Programme. Working Together for Change: Using Person-Centred Information for Commissioning.* London: Department of Health.

Department of Health (2010a) *A Vision for Adult Social Care: Capable Communities and Active Citizens.* London: Department of Health.

Department of Health (2010b) *Personalisation through Person-Centred Planning.* London: Department of Health.

Department of Health (2012) *The Prime Minister's Challenge on Dementia. Delivering Major Improvements in Dementia Care and Research by 2015: A Report on Progress. Challenge.* London: Department of Health.

Gibson, F. (2004) *The Past in the Present: Using Reminiscence in Health and Social Care.* Boston, MA: Health Professionals Press.

Goldsmith, M. (1996) *Hearing the Voice of People with Dementia: Opportunities and Obstacles.* London: Jessica Kingsley Publishers.

Handy, C. (1994) *The Age of Paradox.* Boston, MA: Harvard Business School Press.

HM Government (2012) *Caring for Our Future: Reforming Care and Support.* London: The Stationery Office. Available at www.gov.uk/government/uploads/system/uploads/attachment_data/file/136422/White-Paper-Caring-for-our-future-reforming-care-and-support-PDF-1580K.pdf, accessed on 26 April 2013.

Kitwood, T. (1997) *Dementia Reconsidered: The Person Comes First.* Buckingham: Open University Press.

Kunz, J., Gray, F. and Soltys, F. (2007) *Transformational Reminiscence: Life Story Work.* New York, NY: Springer Publishing Co.

Langer, E. (2009) *Counter-clockwise: Mindful Health and the Power of Possibility.* New York, NY: Ballantine Books.

McKnight, J. (1996) *The Careless Society: Community and Its Counterfeits.* New York, NY: Basic Books.

Marshall, M. (2007) *Living Fuller Lives: The Bamford Review of Mental Health and Learning Disability (Northern Ireland).* Available at www.dhsspsni.gov.uk/living_fuller_lives.pdf, accessed on 26 April 2013.

Mental Health Foundation (2011) *Personalisation and Dementia: A Practitioner's Guide to Self-Directed Support for People Living with Dementia.* London: Mental Health Foundation.

Metcalfe, V. *Living Story Guidance.* Anchor Housing Association, unpublished.

Milwain, E. (2010) 'The brain and person-centred care.' *Journal of Dementia Care 18,* 3, 25–29.

National Institute for Health and Clinical Excellence/Social Care Institute for Excellence (2006) *Supporting People with Dementia and Their Carers in Health and Social Care.* NICE Clinical Guideline 42. London: NICE and SCIE.

Neill, M. and Sanderson, H. (in press) *Circles of Support and Personalisation.* Accessed on www.helensandersonassociates.co.uk.

Nolan, M.R., Davies, S., Brown, J., Keady, J. and Nolan, J. (2004) 'Beyond "person-centred" care: A new vision for gerontological nursing.' *Journal of Clinical Nursing 13,* 3a, 45–53.

Nuffield Council on Bioethics (2009) *Dementia: Ethical Issues.* London: Nuffield Council on Bioethics. Available at www.nuffieldbioethics.org/sites/default/files/Nuffield%20Dementia%20report%20Oct%2009.pdf, accessed on 26 April 2013.

Robertson, J., Emerson, E., Hatton, C., Elliott, J. *et al.* (2005) *The Impact of Person Centred Planning.* Lancaster: Institute for Health Research, Lancaster University.

Sanderson, H. and Lancashire County Council (2010) *Living Well: Thinking and Planning for the End of Your Life.* Stockport: HSA Press.

Sanderson, H. and Lewis, J. (2012) *A Practical Guide to Delivering Personalisation: Person-Centred Practice in Health and Social Care.* London: Jessica Kingsley Publishers.

Sanderson, H. and Miller, R. (in press) *Individual Service Funds at Scale.* London: Jessica Kingsley Publishers.

Schweitzer, P. (ed.) (1998) *Reminiscence in Dementia Care.* London: Age Exchange.

Skills for Care and Dementia UK (2012) *Dementia: Workers and Carers Together: A Guide for Social Care Workers on Supporting Family and Friends Carers of People with Dementia.* Leeds: Skills for Care. Available at www.skillsforcare.org.uk/developing_skills/carers/dementia_workers_and_carers_together.aspx, accessed on 26 April 2013.

Smull, M. and Sanderson, H. (2005) *Essential Lifestyle Planning for Everyone.* Stockport: HSA Press.

Social Care Institute of Excellence (2010) *Personalisation and Mental Capacity.* At a Glance 33 Personalisation Briefing. London: Social Care Institute for Excellence. Available at www.scie.org.uk/publications/ataglance/ataglance33.pdf, accessed on 26 April 2013.

Stirk, S. and Sanderson, H. (2012) *Creating Person-Centred Organisations.* London: Jessica Kingsley Publishers.

Stokes, G. (2010) *And Still the Music Plays: Stories of People with Dementia* (Second Edition). London: Hawker Publications.

Think Local, Act Personal (2011) *Making it Real: Marking Progress Towards Personalised, Community Based Support.* London: TLAP. Available at www.thinklocalactpersonal.org.uk/Latest/Resource/?cid=9091, accessed on 26 April 2013.

Think Local, Act Personal Partnership (2011) *Think Local, Act Personal.* Available at www.thinklocalactpersonal.org.uk, accessed 10 July 2013.

Index